The Frazzled
WORKING WOMAN'S
PRACTICAL GUIDE
TO *Motherhood*

MARY LYON

The
Frazzled
Working Woman's
Practical Guide
to *Motherhood*

MARY LYON

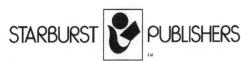

STARBURST PUBLISHERS
™

P.O. Box 4123, Lancaster, Pennsylvania 17604

To schedule Author appearances write:
Author Appearances, Starburst Promotions, P. O. Box 4123
Lancaster, Pennsylvania 17604 or call (717) 293-0939

Credits:
Cover by David Marty Design

The Frazzled Working Woman's Practical Guide To Motherhood

First Printing, October 1997

ISBN: 0-914984-75-6

Library of Congress Catalog Number 97-068723
Printed in the United States of America

Acknowledgments

I have so many people to acknowledge for this book that I'll apologize right now for leaving someone out. I am most grateful to all those who helped and gave me their moral support, or ideas, or places, to park the kids so I could get some work done (like this book)! First of all, to my husband, Bruce, for putting up with me and for helping with absolutely EVERYTHING. And my two little inspirations, of course. And Mom and Dad, I'm grateful more than it's possible to say.

To Grandma (Jo and Jayne), Apa (Goody and Doc), the beloved Jerry Green, Auntie Lockhart Taylor and Carl and Zane, Auntie Leighla and Uncle Dave — Ed and Beau and Nick, Uncle Larry and Aunt Linda, Laurie and John Hartigan, Erin, Caitlin, and ESPECIALLY Tess, Debra and Dave Walker, Katie, and ESPECIALLY Chris, and Jake and Cari.

All of my love to Tom and Linda, Missy and Mimi, Scott and Christine and Cameron, and Tracy and Ron. To Betty Finger and Ruth, Christina and Hank, Lena Sinclair, Julie fallon Steele, Elsa and Cruz, Dean and Amby, Uncle Johnny, Steve and Marty, Adrien Riven, Uncle Mike and Aunt Eve, and Charli.

Deepest thanks to Larry Phillips, Tracy Diestel, and Mike Bassin, plus Barbara, Cindy, Jose and crew.

I am hugely grateful to those souls who suffered this fool gladly, especially June Lockhart, Jim Henson, the one and only Zsa Zsa Gabor, Ann Jillian, Deidra Hall, Kate Mulgrew, Connie Stevens, Jaclyn Smith, Cindy Williams, Susan Dey, and Mary Hart. Extra Appreciation to Lanny Sher, Kitty Felde, Susan Silver, Dave and Sharon Robie, the staff at Starburst Publishers, Gayl Murphy, and Lori De Wall.

Thanks and MANY KIAI's to Keith and Suzanne Hirabayashi Cooke, Mer-Mer Chen, Ali Shah, Mike Bacon, Jeff Wolfe, and Titiana van Hoorn at Champions

Martial Arts. Blessings to Monsignor O'Leary, Father Donie and Cecile Oswald; Charles Shields, Bill Barnes, Jack Walker and Andrea Smith; Richard Preston and Beth Jones; Margo Farrin of Farrin O'Connor Design Studios, and my fellow FIMO-istas.

All my hugs to the world-class folks I love and learned from at the AP, print, photo, and broadcast, both in Los Angeles and Washington. I am honored and grateful to have shared nine years with you. Same for my brothers and sisters in L.A.'s "Radio Mafia," and the friends I still cherish in the general L.A. press corps.

And very special thanks to the late, great Maureen Marten. Sitting in at your funeral Mass made me realize that life's too short, and that it is high time to gather ye rosebuds and additional chapters while ye may.

Dedication

To My husband, editor, and partner-in-life, Bruce Gossard,
and the loves of our lives, Elizabeth and Michael, You are the
inspirations for, and the occasional frustrations behind this book.

If you fail to plan — you can plan to fail.

—Old Entrepreneurial Saying

CONTENTS

Introduction

I did it. I actually won again today. Simply because I survived relatively intact. I think.

This book was born after I began to feel like a mother hen to a number of girlfriends and female colleagues in and around my work place. Women of childbearing age, single, engaged, or already married, who wanted a baby, but still wanted or needed to work. Mainly, they'd wonder how on earth they could handle both. They'd start asking me about that dreamy cliché: "having it all." At first I couldn't see why they were consulting me, but then again, consider the entry-level statistics: married more than 20 years to the same guy, nine years' worth of a MEGA-challenging job capping, all told, roughly a 25-year career in a demanding industry, and two young children — during most of those same, ultra-demanding nine years. Maybe they figured I had the key to the highway.

Well, I don't.

What I have is the key to a long and interesting road with ruts in it. But I also have a set of good, strong tires, a scrappy little engine, and some excellent shock absorbers.

Specifically, what I have is a truckload of ideas and discoveries that I've stumbled upon during the mere act of doing. Short cuts and sanity-savers I learned the hard way, that I sure wish somebody had clued me in about — up front. Primarily about a lot of little things you JUST DON'T THINK ABOUT when it comes right down to rolling up your sleeves and getting into it. Especially if you've never experienced anything like them before, and the only demands you're used to meeting come from the professional world.

And I do mean little things. Sometimes they're almost embarrassingly trivial. But they're the kind of nitpicky details that add up. And I can promise you, if your starship is headed even remotely toward Planet Baby, you won't have time to go back and sift through all the good women's magazines to find the little pearls of wisdom that may or may not apply directly to you.

Becoming pregnant is awfully easy to romanticize. After all, it's usually how you get that way in the first place. And just look at all that darling little baby stuff, and all those adorable, pastel illustrations of kittens, puppies, and storks.

Maybe it's Joan Lunden, Jane Pauley, Demi Moore, or some other high-profile working mom who seems to be pulling it off as terrifically as she looks. Never has a hair out of place, always under control, and seldom stressed. The truth is, these women CAN make it seem easy because they've been at it awhile, probably learned some things the hard way. Let's be honest, they're paid well enough to be able to afford whatever kind of help they might need.

There's also the lore of the pregnant woman as the ultimate beauty. Talk about setting the mood! I've seen lots of visual rhapsodies to modern-day fertility goddesses. My all-time favorite was a bodice-ripper of a painting, with a bulbous heroine reclining languorously on a swan, gliding through poufy clouds, her golden hair streaming behind her like Rapunzel's.

Puh-lease!

Any working woman approaching Planet Baby needs to know what she's REALLY in for. What she'll be taking on — and giving up. It's NOT all pastels. More often than not, it may be poo-poo colored! You mean — you have to get your hands dirty? You better believe it! Hopefully this guide will help you avoid having to get too much else dirty! You're about to become a mother of invention. For better or worse, you're going to have to be.

Chapter 1
Baby: The Ultimate Attitude Adjustment

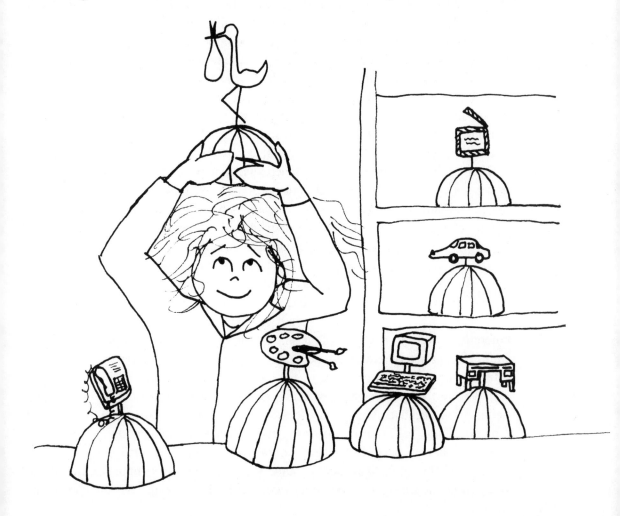

The first reality that pregnancy made me face was that *THERE IS NO SUCH THING AS A SUPERWOMAN*. And you may even have heard this before. Easy to say, but difficult to embrace. And embrace it you must. Repeat this after me 30 times (per minute, maybe), and start getting comfortable with it: *THERE IS NO SUCH THING AS SUPERWOMAN*. If you don't proudly come to live and breathe this, you're setting yourself up for failure, disappointment, and all that other stuff the pop psychologists warn you about. Accept it and move on, and savor what you just did for yourself in the process. You made your load about ten tons lighter.

This became like a "mantra" to me, and helped to reassure me that I wasn't in some decathlon of mothering for which the Gold, Silver and Bronze, and corresponding hurrahs, agents, and athletic shoe endorsements would shortly be awarded. All you need to worry about is how to be the maternal you that you can be.

There's also a larger reality at work here, which may come as a deep-seated jolt to anyone now in the same mind-set I once occupied. See how this strikes you: it's not about YOU anymore. This one marked a real sea-change in me, as a fairly typical child of the '50's and '60's, a daughter of the women's movement, a workaholic type-A personality. This didn't hit me overnight. It sank in slowly. Until my first baby came, it never fully occurred to me that it wouldn't somehow ALWAYS be about me. When my outlook changed, many unexpected bumps in the road I now traveled grew

THERE IS NO SUCH THING AS A SUPERWOMAN.

smoother. You'll be amazed at how this seemingly small inner transformation will improve your outerworld. It will help take away some of your fear about what seems utterly overwhelming right now.

If you're the business-minded type, having a baby is the ultimate merger and acquisition, because someone's about to move in and take over YOU. Look at Connie Chung, for example. After she and Maury Povich adopted their baby boy, you didn't hear a "peep" out of her for quite awhile. This previously single-minded, all-news-all-the-time, dedicated workaholic almost literally went underground. No one saw her storming the Bastille trying to get back on the air after the baby came aboard, did they? Her little one took over completely for a long time. An even swifter takeover than mine managed, for that matter.

That's the way it's SUPPOSED to be, internally speaking, and that change in your focus will be perfectly okay with you soon enough, even if it seems conflicting now. It is an adjustment you may not have anticipated, especially if you've had nothing 'til now but a generous partner or pet with whom to share your center of gravity. If it hasn't overtaken you already, just know that it's enroute. No one *really* made this clear to me.

I never saw this coming. I couldn't imagine having my carefully-planned and ordered life-style co-opted — not by some demanding boss, but by a little squeaker who couldn't even sit up by herself.

Many's the pregnant working woman who seriously presumes she'll have it all back together and be able to return to work within three weeks or so of the baby's arrival. I remember talking to former CNN anchor Bella Shaw about this very subject, and those were her plans, too, when she was pregnant and still on air. She actually wound up stepping away altogether not too long afterwards. Virtually every one of these women comes to realize that the world as she knew it before offspring — has changed completely and forever. Even Madonna has had to admit that, if nothing else, she never could have guessed how much sleep she no longer gets, since her little Lourdes arrived.

I fully expected that three-month maternity leave with Elizabeth would be just fine, and that I'd be anxious to get back to work. I certainly didn't want to be out of the loop for much longer. Too much *unbelievably important stuff* not to be missed was going on with my job. It wasn't long into my maternity leave (maybe a couple of

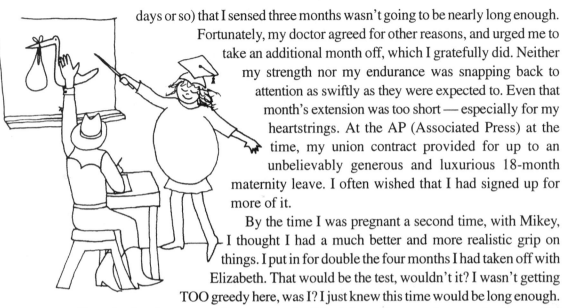

days or so) that I sensed three months wasn't going to be nearly long enough. Fortunately, my doctor agreed for other reasons, and urged me to take an additional month off, which I gratefully did. Neither my strength nor my endurance was snapping back to attention as swiftly as they were expected to. Even that month's extension was too short — especially for my heartstrings. At the AP (Associated Press) at the time, my union contract provided for up to an unbelievably generous and luxurious 18-month maternity leave. I often wished that I had signed up for more of it.

By the time I was pregnant a second time, with Mikey, I thought I had a much better and more realistic grip on things. I put in for double the four months I had taken off with Elizabeth. That would be the test, wouldn't it? I wasn't getting TOO greedy here, was I? I just knew this time would be long enough. Even having been around once already, I hadn't really owned up to the lesson I'd learned with Elizabeth.

I can still remember how my heart sank as I hit the half-way point in that eight-month Maternity leave, and realized I'd be counting more days of leave behind me than ahead of me. People, both inside and outside the business, would say things to me like — "Wow! I'll bet you're anxious to get back to work! Don't you miss it?" And my honest answer would have to be "Well, no." I'd finally accepted that my career-is-my-all attitude had been pre-empted. Something much more important had moved in, and best of all, would love me whether I got that big scoop or not.

I was caught totally by surprise. Believe me, no matter how many board meetings, conventions, or even countries you've run in your career, there's nothing that can prepare you completely for motherhood — either how you feel about it or how you function in it. That old cliché about how babies don't come with instruction manuals is true. (It's also one of my main motivations for writing this book and sharing everything I've learned.)

I wish I'd had something like this to hand to Garth Brooks when I interviewed him at roughly five months into my second pregnancy. That was about three months farther along than his wife, Sandy, was, with their first baby, Taylor Mayne Pearl. When he came into my interview room, I jokingly turned to the side so my stomach profile was even more obvious than usual, and announced — "THIS is what you're in for." Whereupon he grew very serious, and earnestly began to pepper me with questions about what to expect for himself and his wife.

I hope I was helpful. Perhaps my proudest moment was lobbying him to change his mind about not being in the delivery room with his wife. He confessed that he was feeling a bit squeamish about it. (However, he DID go through with it.) And not just that once, but for all three of his children's births.

I wish someone had told ME, because even the savviest of my friends couldn't or didn't have time to tell me everything. I asked Jane Fonda for advice while I was interviewing her for her film *Old Gringo*. She was very kind and sympathetic, and tried to come up with something useful. But she finally conceded that it had been so long since she had her two children that she didn't remember much.

As harrowing, as some of these lessons have been, I still had a walloping good time charting the course to this new land. You may want to keep a journal about it for yourself during your expansion phase. If nothing else, it'll be a wonderful gift to give your child when he or she is old enough to appreciate it.

Let me reassure you of one thing. Because you've come this far in your career, and achieved as much as you have as a professional, you DO have the makings for greatness as a mom. You just need a few real-istic cheat-sheets to shed some light along the way. And you need to know about the attitude

As clueless as you may feel at this point, you're going to be OK.

adjustments ahead — which are quite inevitable and unavoidable. And entirely fitting and proper. You need to know that — as clueless as you may feel at this point, you're going to be OK. You're NOT GOING TO mess it up too badly if you try hard, plan carefully, and your intentions are right.

But motherhood will require, and certainly be worthy of, even more dedication and vigilance than your job does.

I have no degrees or testimonials hanging on my walls. But I do have lots of sweet little photos and finger-paintings. I haven't done any research papers or dissertations on motherhood. I've just lived through it, compared notes with colleagues, and learned from TONS of mistakes! We can let the experts take care of the broader issues and deeper questions. I'm just going to deal with the little stuff. Because I've found that proper management of the little stuff can make the bigger, more important matters a tad easier to deal with. It gives you a sense that at least SOME aspects of your increasingly crazy life can be, and even are, right this minute, controllable by you. And the more you know, the less you'll tear your hair!

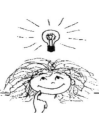

Tips To Remember

✓ Ready for a reality check? When you become a working mom, you're actually talking about a reality CHANGE.

✓ Accept that THERE IS NO SUCH THING AS A SUPERWOMAN, and learn to be okay with that. It will lighten your load and lower the heat on the high expectations you'll have of yourself.

✓ JUST DO YOUR BEST.

✓ Realize that it's not about YOU anymore, anyway, since the baby is really want counts.

✓ This is normal, and will help you come to grips more effectively with your brave new world.

✓ Don't expect for your life to return to what you were used to. The clichés are true — that a baby does indeed change everything. And they don't come with instruction manuals.

✓ Prepare to feel differently about your level of commitment to work, now that you have a child needing you.

✓ Expect to view your life with a new perspective and a new take on unconditional love. Your baby will love you no matter what you do on the job.

✓ Don't worry too much. This is the biggest gig you've ever landed, and yet it will also be fun. Keep a journal about it.

✓ And have confidence in yourself!

Chapter 2

So You're Going To Rock Your Professional Boat

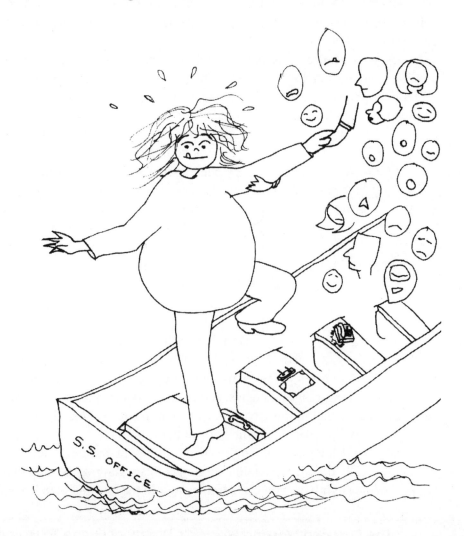

Quick! Before you do ANYTHING else (besides socking away every spare nickel you can get your hands on from this day forward), seek out your company manual or personnel department info or union guidelines. A working woman should enter into pregnancy as fully informed as possible. You need to know what maternity leave policies the company has, compared to what the law now mandates, and what your boss's attitude is about it.

Notify your immediate supervisor first — and as early in your pregnancy as possible. No reason to knock anybody's nose out of joint by violating that all-hallowed chain of command. You can then ask him or her to recommend whom you tell next, and how, and what to do after that. Inviting your supervisor in at the front of the line is a subtle way of encouraging a potential ally who may be able to run a phenomenal amount of interference for you later on. He or she will appreciate as much advance notice as you can provide, especially the "first" advance notice. Frankly, it's just simple courtesy.

Same thing goes for everyone else at the office, once they, too, have been integrated into the early-warning system. It lets *them* plan ahead, as well.

Be as helpful and accommodating as you can. Very early in your pregnancy is when you can pitch in a bit more, offer a few extra hours, design some contingency plans or long-range strategies, and burnish your image as a real trouper they value and realize they'll miss. Now is when you'll still feel like doing so, and you won't have any little person needing you at home — YET.

I recommend this, even if you're in the throes of morning sickness. Which sometimes really does happen in the mornings. If so, you may be able to rearrange your schedule slightly so you can come in later in the day and then leave later. Or maybe you could suggest an adjusted week, four 10-hour days instead of five 8-hour ones or something like that. I recommend that, if at all possible, you avoid burning up sick days when morning sickness strikes. Unless, of course, you're truly suffering. You'll look like even MORE of a trouper while working through it. Besides, you could need a sick day for a very fatiguing day close to the end when you'll be your largest and most strained. Or you might want to backload those precious sick days into your maternity leave.

Miserable as it is, morning sickness doesn't last, and you WILL survive it. You should check with your doctor if you have any questions, but chances are good that this phase will pass long before your waistline and most of your energy starts to. Or, hopefully, you'll luck out like I did (both times, thank God!) and you won't have any. But if you do, soldier on to the best of your ability (with your handy supply of soda crackers nearby) while still in the first trimester or two. I can assure you that you won't be in any shape or mood for it later on.

Investigate how many ways beyond the banking of sick days you can reasonably extend your leave. Whether you can add on your vacation, personal days, or any other time off that you're allowed. This should be figured out in advance, and your personnel people can help you with it. Once you're out on maternity leave, you may wish you had twice the time you arranged for. Your doctor could very well decree that for you.

Offer to recruit your own maternity leave replacement. That may help smooth the transition and ease your increasingly harried mind a little. If that person is already on your team, he or she may not have a hidden agenda to promote at your expense, and can keep you tapped into the office grapevine so you won't miss too much while you're away. But keep your eyes wide open about this, too. It's unfortunate, but true, that even the sweetest souls with the best intentions are capable of changes of heart — especially after they've had a taste of your gig for awhile. That's why it's very important, while you're still there, to go as all out as you can stand to.

Check, in advance, whether or not you're expected to train your replacement. This didn't occur to me the first time around, when I was totally out of the loop. My fill-in was chosen by my supervisor from outside L.A. That meant she had the additional job of relocating in order to take this assignment. She was a woman I'd never met, but whom he knew well. Therefore, I operated under the belief that everything, except sharing the phone numbers and tips she'd need, was out of my hands. No one clued me in about this, and I didn't realize I should have spoken up about it. And, believe me, if only I'd known, I would have gladly moved heaven and earth to do WHATEVER was needed.

Check, in advance, whether or not you're expected to train your replacement.

In the meantime, my workload grew as swollen as my belly, especially in those last couple of months when I had to struggle mightily to weather both. My supervisor, too, was busy. Soon I was at T-minus two weeks and counting. By then, I was hunkered down on an extremely demanding story — the long-running saga of Zsa Zsa Gabor versus the Beverly Hills Police Department.

I had no time to reach my replacement to set up a transition meeting, and no one told me when she'd be formally installed — no less fully moved in. I felt badly, too, because she deserved much more than a few hurried phone calls from me, which was all I could manage. So, at the last minute, there was a mad scramble, with extra money needing to be shelled out for my supervisor's airfare and hotel room while he came out from Washington to shepherd her through it.

What's worse, news of his annoyance got back to me second — and third— hand, and years later, too — while I was out on my second maternity leave, no less. Which meant I had something extra to worry about and divert my attention while I was in a position to do nothing about it. A bad taste in your supervisor's mouth, even one you didn't realize was there, or intend to leave there, can last a long time. Believe me, this is a trap you DON'T want to fall into, or find yourself pushed into.

By the time I was about to take out on my second maternity leave, I HAD recruited my own replacement. She lived in the same city and was easier to reach by phone. We'd arranged to spend most of my last week together, either at night in the bureau, learning the "nuts and bolts," or during the day, when she went along with me on assignment.

One of those assignments was a late afternoon-early evening one which covered the Academy of Country Music Awards show. As it turned out, that was also the night when the 1992 L.A. riots began.

I realized this would not be the usual awards show coverage because about half the regular reporters were absent from the backstage press area. (They'd been reassigned to cover the first Rodney King trial verdict.) I remember the ordinarily jaunty cameraman from "Entertainment Tonight," had an uncharacteristically serious expression on his face as he talked on a cell phone to his assignment desk while the awards ceremoney went on. He quickly alerted the rest of us that rioting had broken out in town.

Suddenly, the bright and festive atmosphere backstage turned heavy and dour.

Suddenly, the bright and festive atmosphere backstage turned heavy and dour. I checked with my own assignment desk in Washington where they informed me that they didn't need me to divert to "riot duty." I should stay with what I was doing, because the hard-news reporters had the riots well-covered. So, I concentrated on the event at hand, and helped my replacement get her "sea-legs" strictly on the entertainment beat.

By the time it was over, in an uneasy silence, we carpooled back to the bureau through the smell, haze, and anger of the smoke and fires burning through numerous inner-city neighborhoods. We were not sure what lay ahead for either of us. The bureau was boiling with activity as more and more reporters were called in to cover this cataclysmic developing story. Our bureau, just a few blocks from City Hall, reeked of the smoke.

And with all hell breaking loose around me, I was fighting to stay focused on editing tape of happy country music stars with all the new awards they'd worked and hoped so hard for. On a night like this, Heaven only knew when any of the awards would get on the air.

Needless to say, it was *another* very long evening, trying to get the work done and *then* trying to feed it all in, when the folks in Washington were much more concerned (and understandably so) about getting "hot stuff," ASAP, from the riot zones.

The next day the fires were still burning furiously, and the whole city was on alert. It was a Thursday, and I had one more day to go before maternity leave. My husband was beside himself with fear for me (and our future son) downtown, so near the thick of things — especially in the shape I was in. So much so that when he woke me up late that morning (again I'd pre-arranged to start the day later, anticipating a later evening finish), he announced that I wouldn't be going in to work that day. I could work from home, he declared.

I was so exhausted and stressed, just on general principles — no less because of what was happening in the news — that I didn't feel up to fighting it. Besides, Lorrie Morgan's publicist had left word at the office that my one appointment of the day, an afternoon interview with Lorrie, had been canceled. She'd seen the news coverage of what was going on around L.A. and decided to head back to Nashville.

The bureau had also become a victim of overcrowding, as even more reporters (including many from affiliated newspapers) had moved in on every spare computer terminal, making it THEIR headquarters. There wasn't any extra room, particularly for an extraneous someone like me who wasn't even on that beat to begin with. I figured I was probably doing them a favor by staying out of their hair. (Especially since I wouldn't be able to get out of anybody's way quickly, moving as slowly and painfully as I was!)

So, before I even struggled out of bed, I called Washington to let them know.

My husband Bruce, the computer whiz, worked with my Washington editor to hook my computer into the AP system. I then researched, wrote and filed everything that was needed. I already had interview tape which I packaged with the equipment I always kept with me. Then I fed everything to Washington over a special phone Bruce had rewired for me, that which afforded a much better sound quality. The folks who took in my material expressed surprise and pleasure at how I didn't miss a beat with any of my job responsibilities — even when not going near the bureau. My replacement-in-training reported being delighted with the welcome spare day in which to wrap up lots of things on her end. And all's well that ends well.

NOT!!!!!!

It turned out that my supervisor wasn't exactly overjoyed that I hadn't valiantly tempted fate and had gone downtown to the bureau to work as usual. My press tags would have gotten me safely through ANY police lines or riot zones, he reasoned. There was no excuse, (even though I pulled a full workload that day, counting all the phone calls I routinely made from home). Not only that, but neither were they impressed one level up the management food chain. I was later told that one individual in particular, was miffed to the gills that I'd worked from home that day. Absolutely no reason for it! And I hadn't given enough advance notice! (As if anyone can predict such a calamitous turn of events in the first place.)

I've known working women who've discovered midstream, or after they've returned to work from maternity leave, that there were leftover hard feelings at upper levels in the office. Therefore, it's a good idea to document all the steps you take beforehand, all the "notice" you've given, plans you've implemented, extra work hours you've put in, the reasons for it, what you accomplished, and the contingencies you've thought through. Hopefully, you won't need to show any of this at a later date. But you'll be grateful that you did if you sense there may be complications. That way you'll be able to prove that you went by the book, and quite likely far beyond it, on the company's behalf; AND that the company's cause was not compromised in any way.

My supervisor, on the other hand, did have his moments of absolutely inspired enlightenment. The best example of this came with the Oscars of 1992, just two short months before I was to bail out for Mikey's birth. It was also the season of *Basic Instinct* — which had spawned many objections from the gay community about the way gays were portrayed onscreen. That particular Oscar day, one radical group had been expected to stage a noisy and rather eye-catching in-your-face protest just outside the event.

Since my supervisor usually was busy hooking up all our phone and broadcast loop connections in the backstage press area, and coordinating last-minute details with the assignment desk in Washington, it often fell to me to go outside and investigate what else might be going on that would be newsworthy. This time, however, he gave himself that assignment, noting the difficulty he guessed I'd have because of my "condition," and without any snide remarks, I might add. Not to mention the truly incongruous images that might result if I went out there looking and feeling as I did. So I gratefully stayed behind, inside, minding all our phones and equipment at our assigned seats, while there were still a few empty chairs available on which to prop up my swollen legs.

Think and plan carefully for ALL the added expenses. Especially insurance coverage while you're out.

Think and plan carefully for ALL the added expenses. Especially insurance coverage while you're out. Will you still be on active status (and thus, covered) or inactive status (and thus, quite exorbitantly UNcovered)? Does your mate have enough insurance to cover you and the new arrival? Will you have to buy more, look elsewhere, or do as I had to — and pay the company monthly (through the nose) to stay covered until I could return to active duty and to automatic coverage again?

You'll also be shelling it out for diapers (either store-bought or a service), laundry, food, photos, clothes, baby equipment, and scads of surprises. Like the two days of phototherapy for Mikey, whose little system needed jump-starting in a special light booth to keep him from developing jaundice when he was less than a week old! Kiss a fast couple of thousand bucks good-bye on that one! At times it will feel as if you're "hemorrhaging money."

Will you get — and do you really expect you'll want — your old job back? Think about this long and hard. Flex-time, part-time, or job-sharing options may suddenly become appealing for easing back into the job. Telecommuting and teleconferencing are gaining ground in some of the more forward-thinking companies. If your company doesn't have any such policies and you feel like being assertive, perhaps you can initiate them yourself. You may face the so-called "Mommy-track," where women with children in a corporate setting risk being shifted to paths that don't lead to upper-management positions — while their "unencumbered" childless sisters stay on the fast track toward the top.

By the time your baby comes and revolutionizes your universe, you may find that's exactly how you want it. You may soon realize you'd rather be an upper-level mother than an upper-level manager. Believe it or not, these course changes DO happen. If they start happening to you, I'd like to reassure you that it doesn't mean you've sold out on any commitment to career excellence. It's simply that you've just received a different form of job upgrade!

Find out how long before your due date that you can close down, for financial reasons of course, and also, for plain ol' practical reasons. Believe me, by the time you're pushing eight months — and an amazing increase of weight and mass —

you'll be anxious to get out of the fray, put your feet up, and stay that way. I found it awkward and sometimes downright painful merely to walk. My first pregnancy plunged me into my own personal *Waterworld*. My second one did likewise. Fifty extra pounds of fluid and fetal weight, both times, made me look like the Michelin Tire Man.

But even as brutally honest as I'm trying to be about all this, I won't divulge the final readings on my bathroom scale on the day each of my kids was born. After all, my mother is gonna read this!

I guess all of that inflation during both pregnancies was cosmic payback for having no morning sickness.

Prepare to move your wedding ring or other significant bauble from your ring finger to your pinkie, or maybe to a chain around your neck. You'll still look married if your boss or some client has a hang-up about such things, and you won't have to have the ring cut off, as I did, when I waited too long and my ring finger began to look as though it were pregnant all by itself.

At one point toward the end, I was so bloated that I felt like a water balloon. I suddenly understood the true meaning behind that old cliché about being "barefoot and pregnant." My feet were so swollen I literally popped out of my shoes. The two remaining pairs of comfortable, low-heeled pumps I'd come to rely upon had to be permanently retired, because I had actually ripped through the leather and the stitching along the edges. My legs! Inflated to such an extreme that I could poke a finger into the skin and the indentation would stay intact for more than a minute before the fluids oozed back in to fill it out.

This became uncomfortably apparent during the Zsa Zsa Gabor cop-slapping trial in Beverly Hills, when I discovered several uncomfortable things, come to think of it. I wound up sitting on the marble floor of the courthouse hallways a lot. The press was everywhere. You had to arrive at least an hour before court opened in order to get a place to patch in all your audio and video cables, and if you were lucky, a seat on the benches along the walls for yourself. I, of course, needed about double the average space, for all my radio equipment, and also for ME!

There were many times when some kind reporter pal or technician or someone would give up their seat so I could sit down. Bless them! But there was one cameraman who held his turf and gave up only a sneer when I asked for help. Be ready for that. Not *everyone* you run into will be sympathetic and helpful.

When I had to resort to the floor, I'd be aghast whenever I'd change position. Whichever side of my leg was pressed against the floor came to look precisely as though it HAD been pressed against the floor. For several minutes, it would be as FLAT as the floor, until the excess fluid inflated it again.

This was, of course, after I had managed to hoist myself up onto my feet again. That always took longer, because there was so much extra bulk to me to begin with. So, whenever Zsa Zsa or some attorney of interest exited the courtroom and we all had to give chase to get our mikes in their faces, I had to practically roll myself into place. Again, taking up two reporters' worth of space in the process. No one ever laughed, bless their hearts! The press corps covering the Zsa Zsa affair was undoubtedly used to seeing me lumbering along, gargantuan belly leading the way, equipment caddie taking up the rear. They probably regarded me as the case mascot or something.

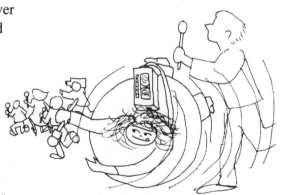

Even funnier than the vision of me there was the day there were two of us. An equally pregnant City News Service reporter took the Zsa Zsa beat for the day, and we found each other! How could we help it? The place started to look like a watermelon convention.

Consider bailing out a week before you'd actually planned to. That's because the stork may decide not to coordinate schedules with you. I sure wish I'd allowed myself a little more time before Elizabeth came. I really could have used it.

The day of the Zsa Zsa trial verdict — a huge news day for me as an entertainment reporter — was the last day before my scheduled maternity leave. It was the last Friday in September, and my due date was October 15th. Looked good on paper, anyway. However, I was rushed by my doctor into the maternity ward the following Wednesday afternoon! Perhaps it was the stress of the event, the deadline pressure, all that courtroom and press conference tape to cut and package, or something, shaking up my system and zipping me into fast-forward mode. You suppose my daughter was in a hurry to get outside to meet Zsa Zsa? Then again, it could just be the effect Zsa Zsa has on some people!

Zsa Zsa did pat my belly at one point during a lunch break and ask if I planned to name it after her.

That was some day! Friends who had to work on weekends had set up my baby shower for that Friday lunch time, and a colleague at the courthouse had agreed to beep me if it looked as if a verdict was imminent. I had planned to start my day late, because I knew I was in for a long night, regardless of what happened. The beeper went off several times during the course of lunch (which I never did get to eat). The final time, it was for real, and everyone there had to race out to the parking lot with me, throwing baby gifts and haphazardly wrapped sandwiches into my car so I could make it to the courthouse on time. Fortunately, I'd advised everyone at the beginning that this COULD happen, and apologized in advance. A good reporter never forgets the disclaimer!

Pregnant women in the advanced stages waddle when they walk, which may make you feel a little silly. You'll start feeling like you have a coconut in your crotch. That's no coconut. It's the baby's head, settling into the pelvic bone like an egg in an egg cup. Your powers of concentration will be diverted from your job to how you're feeling. You will lumber through the office more slowly because there's more of you to move around, and it's a much greater effort to do so.

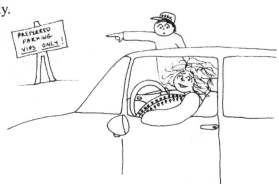

One thing I heartily recommend, which may sound mighty nit-picky, is something I usually forgot to do, and always kicked myself for, afterwards. Don't you fall into this trap, too. If you've got an appointment somewhere, if it's AT ALL in unfamiliar territory, ask the person on the other end of the phone if it involves climbing stairs!!! Man oh man, will you hate every upward step you have to conquer as you grow bigger and bigger. The strain on your legs and lungs and heart will leave you wheezing and perspiring by the time you reach the top step. And what a cool, collected, professional image THAT's bound to convey!

I can remember interviews with Mary Hart, Jon Lovitz, and "Young Indiana Jones" star, Sean Patrick Flanery — all second-story acts — during which the first several minutes of our meetings were more or less a waste. That's because, in each case, I'd be groaning and gasping by the time I'd heave my heavy bulk up long flights of stairs to reach them. It also took much longer than I'd expected to regain my composure and any semblance of normal breathing before I could actually begin the interviews.

I was such a mess eight months before Mikey's arrival. While struggling to reach Sean Patrick Flanery I think I actually frightened him. He was, after all, a very young man, and the way his eyes bugged out and the color faded from his face when he first saw me, I got the feeling that he'd never had a close encounter with as huge a pregnant woman as I was. Fortunately, I'd reached the point at which I'd long since given up being embarrassed about anything.

Same strategy applies if it's simply a longer walk to get where you need to go rather than climb stairs. I found that, at some studios, the guards at the front gate were very sympathetic and helpful to me when I drove up and appealed to them to let me park at least a "wee bit" closer than usual. All they ever had to do (which wasn't difficult) was to look a little more closely into my car. My stomach was hard to miss. I'll always be grateful to the parking lot attendant at the Pasadena Civic Auditorium that one late summer, when I had to go cover the Emmys. Yes, I had pre-arranged press parking. But this wonderful man let me in to an even more exclusive section after he saw how close I was to needing a second parking place for the stork.

Of course, I appreciated folks like this even more, after staggering through walks that went on for blocks when I was on the way to an interview at a studio. Naturally, my appointments on the set of "The Arsenio Hall Show" or "L.A. Law" were across the lot from visitor parking.

That's one reason why I will always fondly regard Susan Dey, with whom I had an interview just a few weeks before Elizabeth arrived. Susan refused to begin our meeting until she had brought me a cold drink, positioned me just so on the sofa, and propped my swollen feet up on the table for me.

Be prepared to feel a little "homely." Over and over I heard about how beautiful pregnant women are. How they glow. You actually might feel that way, which I heartily applaud, not to mention envy! Many women do. But I was not one of them. Besides, there's nothing like reaching the stage where you suddenly realize that's one WHALE of a stomach blooming just below your rib cage — and having to report on Hugh Hefner and his gorgeously-curved then-fiancee, Kimberley Conrad, who had also previously appeared as *Playboy* readers' "Playmate of the Year." If I didn't already have a complex about the way I looked, I sure did by the end of THAT assignment.

Over and over I tried to take it to heart about how lovely I supposedly was in this condition. And over and over I found I didn't believe a word of it. Especially when I looked in the mirror. I felt fat, fatter, and fattest. I knew that however I dressed, I would never be able to hide my largesse, especially because, on me, it went from stem to stern. After a while, I sort of threw up my hands and accepted it, knowing it would be temporary, and that this was one of the only times in my life where I WASN'T SUPPOSED TO HAVE A WAISTLINE! And once I did accept that, did I EVER feel liberated! After a lifetime of dieting and self-denial, I decided I had earned the right to let up just a little bit.

Right about then, I recalled an item in some magazine quoting Christie Brinkley as saying that, while she was pregnant with her daughter Alexa, she allowed herself the occasional forbidden figure-defying luxury of peanut butter. I remember how she'd said she figured she was entitled to it in those circumstances. And this boosted my morale as I, too, dove into the Skippy. Yep, it's you and me, Christie, two sisters in pregnancy shoulder-to-shoulder together down in the bowels of that peanut butter jar to the bitter end! Well, of course she snapped back into shape MUCH quicker than I ever could have. (I didn't have nearly the shape she did to start with.) When I later saw her while covering a City Hall event, I asked her about that. And she said she didn't remember ever making any such a statement.

Rachel Hunter certainly remembered. Not about scarfing down the peanut butter per se, but certainly about sinning at the dinner table. She clearly recalled thinking that since both her pregnancies were such a small part of her life — then why not? She explained to me that she actually enjoyed seeing her stomach go out and having a huge lump in the front, watching her concave curves grow outrageously convex in pregnancy, and not being able to see her feet anymore. Being on the beach with husband Rod Stewart, both of them deliriously happy about the child they were making together, and studying the area where her belly button used to be with the greatest fascination.

She also admitted, that even though she got rid of her 30-pound weight gain after daughter Renee was born, and 35 pounds after son Liam arrived, her body was never quite the same. She found, as I have, that her ribcage had permanently expanded, after stretching to accommodate two babies. Many women discover that their feet have gained a size. I had to get a new wedding ring because the one that had to be cut off and soldered together again while I was pregnant with Elizabeth wouldn't go back over my knuckle anymore.

But even feeling the way I did about how I looked, I could still find some beauty in my pregnant state. My consolation during this time was a set of fingernails almost completely transformed, and hair that appeared to have doubled in bulk. As you'll notice yourself, all those extra vitamins and meals fortified with calcium and protein will leave them as buff as can be. Besides, your body's *really into* doing right by such items right now. Enjoy this while it lasts. After you've had the baby and breast-feeding's tapered off, you'll find your soft, peely, breaky nails returning, and all that fabulous new growth of hair falling out in handfuls. Yep, some things really ARE too good to be true.

Other things will be just plain odd. You may start to smell different. Maybe a little like heated milk or butter. Your added weight and girth means you're apt to sweat more, which will compound this condition. In my case it wasn't an unpleasant smell, it was just odd. No one (even those closest to me) ever mentioned this, so perhaps it wasn't noticeable to others. But I certainly was conscious of it.

One of the first times I became aware of this was while crouched at the feet of Michael Keaton, straining to hold my mike in proper position in front of his face to get decent audio quality out of a large group interview with him for the first *Batman* movie.

It was the first time I'd tried a new style of pregnancy outfit called a "slip dress" — with a generously-cut skirt attached to the bottom of a long, sheer, lingerie-style tank-top with another generously-cut overshirt covering it. I soon discovered that if you moved, or stretched, or strained even a little bit, the overshirt soon wouldn't be covering what it was supposed to, nor would the hem of the skirt. I battled a constant dilemma all through the interview, how close could I afford to come to Keaton's face and still get good-quality soundbites, keep track of the course of the questions and answers, get my questions in there, *and* make sure I remained sartorially secure.

I've always been more sensitive to heat and crowding, and crowding is certainly what we were forced to do around Michael Keaton. It made me feel uncomfortably warm to the point of working up a sweat, and then I *knew* I didn't want to be any closer to him or anyone else than I absolutely had to be.

I can recall often feeling tremendously self-conscious about this. Because, toward the end of both my pregnancies, almost *anything* I did, beyond batting my eyelashes, worked up a sweat. I came to dread crowded press conferences when slews of reporters and camera crews are together in close quarters, all clamoring for the same objective.

I painfully remember having to stand for hours in a packed Rodeo Drive gallery for an exhibition of Sylvester Stallone's paintings. I'd tried to get there early, so if he had a moment, he could quickly take care of my interview needs. After all, as a radio reporter I had only a small microphone and tape recorder — not a crew full of technicians with equipment and lighting to mess with.

As the room grew more and more jammed, heated, and more crowded with camera crews, I was pressed into a little corner. Everyone was taken care of before me, by a slew of slim and elegant young gallery women who I suspected had probably never been pregnant. I finally got my turn after hinting to them that, if I had to wait around on my feet any longer in the heat and congestion, I feared that I'd pass out right in front of everyone and the other reporters would have a new story to cover instead of Stallone.

You WILL be tired. Let me tell you how tired! You won't be able to get a decent night's sleep because as your stomach expands, you'll find it more difficult to achieve a comfortable position. All that baby and fluid and other stuff in there will be crowding against your leg nerves and blood vessels, your bladder, and lungs. The simple act of breathing will be awkward toward the end. Soooooo, you'll be sleep-deprived during the day. And yes, of course, that means when you're on duty.

I can't count how many screenings I attended, for the sake of interviewing the cast the next day, which I never saw all the way through because I dozed off in the middle of them. Same thing for celebrity press conferences, set up by various networks to hype new TV shows. I think I've fallen asleep on some of the best of 'em. Arnold Schwarzenegger, Sidney Poitier, George Lucas, John Cusack, and Ione Skye. Kevin Bacon and Elizabeth Perkins, Willem Dafoe and Mickey Rourke, Woody Harrelson and Wesley Snipes are just a few of the celebrities I owe apologies to on *that* score!

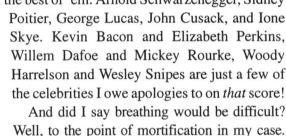

And did I say breathing would be difficult? Well, to the point of mortification in my case. Because in several of these, I wouldn't merely fall asleep with my head tilted against the back of my chair. I'd snore, sometimes loudly. I'm surprised no one ever asked me to leave. Maybe they thought I was more entertaining than whatever movie we were screening at the moment.

Your back WILL ache. So will your joints, as they soften and expand. Your whole body is doing this so the critical inside part of you that needs to let the baby through will be loose enough to do so. I wish I could say the same about the outside of me. The skin of my legs and feet actually stung because the bloating within caused it to stretch so extremely. It became tight, shiny, and very bizarre-looking.

Realities like these, plus hormonal changes and furious chemical reactions inside you, added to your nonstop worrying about what lies ahead, WILL leave you grouchy and much more emotional than usual. Expect this and plan for it. Particularly if you have a lot of paperwork or equipment to carry in and out of the office every day. I found that, within a few months of my delivery date, I had to invest in one of those little collapsible flight-attendant caddies on wheels. It made a huge difference. Every so often you may also want to treat yourself to an hour with a masseuse for your aching back. A splendid idea! But be sure to get a referral from your obstetrician or birthing center. All masseuses are not alike, and a pregnant client requires specialized skill.

Finally, if you ARE going to be firing right back up on full throttle after your maternity leave is over, as opposed to tip-toeing back to work on a scaled-back schedule, be prepared to be *incredibly* disoriented. Maybe even a little despondent. It's likely you will have grown very accustomed to your mellow new life at home, looking after and bonding with the wee one. There will be a RADICAL difference in the stress factor. My first interview just days after my first maternity leave was over couldn't have been more appropriate: Eric Pierpoint, who played the extra-terrestrial cop in the TV series "Aliennation." After all, I was feeling pretty alien by then, myself.

My first day back after both job leaves was on the first working day of February. In both instances, it was because I wanted to be back in the saddle and reacclimated to work before the Oscar nominations — that usually are held around Valentine's Day. This is the famous event that's alive and kicking at 5:35 a.m. Pacific time, because one of the suits at the Academy of Motion Picture Arts and Sciences decided it would be really neat-o to have the nominations announced live on all the morning shows like "Today" and "Good Morning America" — on THEIR east coast scheduling.

Invariably, my "litttle one" had bad dreams or restless slumbers the night before and needed my comforting after hours, despite my desperate attempts to get to bed no later than 8:00 p.m. (since I had to be up and on duty by 3:30 a.m.)! Invariably, the movies most likely to be nominated were all released while I was away on leave and not going to that many screenings. So I had to research like crazy and play as aggressive a game of catch-up as I could whenever I had the chance. Once the high drama and suspense of who got what nominations was over, I had to high-tail it back across town to the bureau to start calling the nominees for reaction, but fast. Talk about going from 0 to 60!

Oscar nomination day was always one of the key events of the year and demanded all my attention and endurance. It was like running a marathon. It always required oodles of overtime, and by the time I had rounded the bend past about noon (when my urgent deadlines had passed) and there was no more phone calling or react chasing to do, I was always totally "fried" from being on tension overdrive, and my lack of sleep was rapidly catching up with me. Plus, I still had several hours worth of mop-up work to do for the next day.

Then, late in the afternoon I'd stumble home, bleary-eyed, hoping that in my altered state of consciousness I hadn't forgotten anything. And I knew I wouldn't be in any position to go right to bed when I got home. Elizabeth would be needing me, and I her, and of course after Mikey was here, too, that would be true for them BOTH.

After Mikey's birth, as well, I returned to work on February first, and was promptly greeted with a big assignment to be covered — not midmonth with the Oscars, but much sooner. Like the next day. This time, it was the Soul Train Awards

---

nominations, involving an area of music in which I wasn't exactly an expert. Here again, I had to research like mad, and hope for the best the next day, as I hurried to the story, praying that I still remembered how to do this, and where and how to patch everything together for the sake of good audio! Remember, I had been out on a much longer leave with Mikey, and was sure that my skills were rusty.

It was just luck, and maybe the indulgence of the R'n'B/Urban angel that I waded in, a little ahead of schedule, found all the right equipment plug-ins, had some time to study the press kit, and then cover the story.

I also managed to pull aside the women of En Vogue for a brief one-on-one interview, since they were there reading the nominations, and pleasantly surprised to be reading off their own names on a few of the categories. Might as well grab 'em if I get a chance to, I thought. I wasn't sure about the most recent details of their background, whether they'd gotten married or divorced or how many hits they'd had in the past (especially while I was out of the loop), but they were charming and enthusiastic, and I did get some very acceptable material to use for soundbites.

Well, that was nice. Only later did I learn that our R'n'B/Urban editor back in Washington was eager to get tape of them, especially, and the material I'd just brought in with only half a clue was exactly what he'd hoped for and more. Sometimes someone up there decides to give you a break and sing in harmony with you when you thought you'd be stuck doing a solo.

Tips 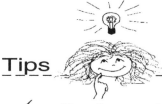 To Remember

✓ Your first step should be to notify the people at work. ALWAYS starting with your immediate supervisor. This is both courteous and wise, and is liable to make things easier for you.

✓ Give everyone as much advance notice as possible, and then really dive in as a team player. Doing as much extra, EARLY ON (especially as it applies to maintaining the job while you're gone) will help your coworkers and yourself. Even if you have morning sickness. Morning sickness doesn't last. Besides, you won't feel up to it later on.

✓ Figure out the in's and out's of your maternity leave, backload it with your leftover vacation time and sick days if you can, and go for the longest leave you can get. Expect to underestimate your wish to stay at home with the baby.

✓ Find out if you can recruit your replacement, and if you have to train anyone.

✓ Document everything you've done above and beyond the call of duty, just in case.

✓ Check the status of your insurance coverage while you're away, and what you may have to do about it.

✓ Prepare to spend money. Lots of it. In greater and greater amounts. And it'll last for years!

✓ The inner changes you'll experience as a working mom are worth a great deal of thought. And they're the cause of some VERY UNEXPECTED new adventures.

✓ You may want to rethink your single-minded career pursuits, either partially or totally. And there are options available: Like flex-time, part-time, telecommuting and job-sharing. Consider starting such policies at work if there are none currently in effect. It may startle you most to realize that this change of direction is okay, and not at all uncommon.

✓ Equally startling external changes abound when you're pregnant: Weight and water gain — sometimes in huge amounts. Swelling, achy joints, painful extremities, an odd way of walking, more sweating and odd smells, self-consciousness, and difficulty breathing, sleeping, and concentrating, but who's counting!

✓ You may feel awkward and a little homely. AND TIRED! AND GRUMPY!

✓ Take comfort in the facts you have to face: You're not SUPPOSED to have a waistline, so go ahead and eat well, and focus on nourishing your new little sprout. And it happens to every woman this way. Besides, there's not One Thing you can do about it.

✓ Your body may change permanently — as in size of waist, hips, fingers, or feet. But for awhile, at least, enjoy your newly resurrected hair and nails!

✓ Expect to feel a little disoriented, and perhaps despondent once you return to work. Also be prepared for the stress level to rise exponentially!

Chapter 3

My Own "Big Tent" Theory

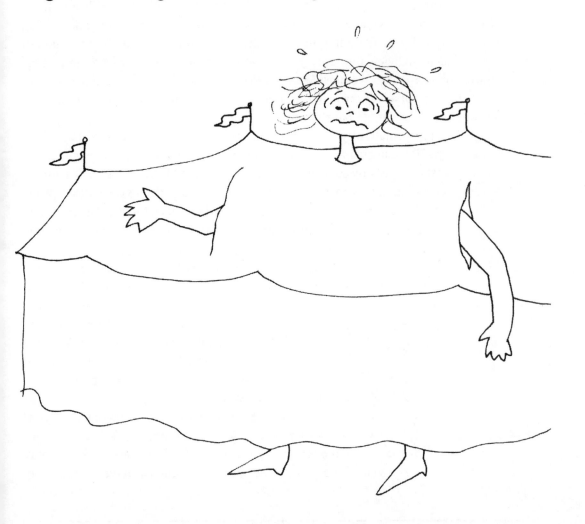

For all he had to say about a big tent philosophy, the late politician Lee Atwater never knew the half of it. We women who've worked while we're "fruiting," on the other hand, do. And all too well.

Work clothes while pregnant must be chosen with ruthless clear-headedness. After all, we civilians can't use the tricks available to a pregnant actress: disguising that bulging belly by holding pillows or jackets in front of it, standing behind tall chairs, and being viewable only in close-up. Our main concerns are aesthetics, comfort, and ease of movement. We want to be sufficiently attractive and well-constructed to see ourselves through the largeness of pregnancy plus however long it'll take our bodies to deflate back to normal, or near normal size.

By now, many maternity shops cater to working women who need to look as though they still mean business as they become human "balloons." But what I never could understand was why so many styles are in horizontal stripes and wild patterns that only accentuate what I'm trying to conceal. Plus, many florals or "cutesy" prints will distract from the professional look I want. Maternity clothes, if they're any good at all, will be fairly expensive. And most of them will serve you for just a few months out of your life.

And, as I noted earlier, with the slip-skirt affair at the *Batman* junket, they may not be constructed appropriately enough for what YOU need to be doing in your job. Are they really built to take the punishment you'll be dishing out on an average day? Will they accommodate different kinds of movement? And/or positioning? And heft of body-weight and/or breast-weight?

It would be better to reassess what's in your closet already to see what might work. You'll yearn for the tent-dress craze of a few seasons back and may want to haul your old one out if you still have it and it's in good shape. If you were into the baggy "Annie Hall" look years ago, that might be worth revisiting.

You'll come to appreciate tunics more than ever before — they're ideal, both now and later. Stick to single color themes, since that helps draw the eye up and down rather than sideways. Long vests, scarves, and necklaces also add welcome vertical lines to offset your expansion. Big shirts and boyfriend jackets — that came from the back of your man — are also good. The boyfriend jackets that you may already have in your closet may still fit, but probably weren't cut roomy enough to accommodate you now. Blouson-style dresses and overshirts are also worth trying because they're pouchy by nature and are more fitted below the belly.

You'll find you may actually enjoy pregnancy dressing if you let your imagination go out dancing a little.

Comfortable shoes are essential, and as the pregnancy progresses, the flatter the heels are, the better.

For more formal needs, like the Academy Awards ceremony I covered two months before Mikey's arrival, I stumbled upon an absolutely sensational approach that made many of my non-pregnant women colleagues (even the ones with the enviably teeny waistlines) sit up and take notice. I recommend it enthusiastically, because it works like a dream, whether you're pregnant or not. And you're guaranteed not to see the same thing on someone else — regardless of the occasion.

I found a magnificent, full-length antique kimono, in flowing black fabric with gold embroidery, in the corner of some off-the-beaten-path boutique. It wasn't all that expensive. I wore it over a plain black shirt and trousers. Despite my size, all you saw was the beautiful thing I had draped myself with, and I actually looked quite good. It was so flattering that I wound up wearing that same outfit again and again, long after my baby-making days were over.

You'll find you may actually enjoy pregnancy-dressing if you let your imagination go out dancing a little. This is the time to experiment with more unconventional things, one-of-a-kind wearable art, and wonderful ethnic designs in import and specialty shops here and there. Jackets, overshirts, trousers, and caftans from India, Central America, and Africa, in hand-dyed and embellished fabrics, are to die for anyway, and are almost always cut generously. They're usually *quite* reasonably priced. Perfect for pregnancy AND post-pregnancy dressing, not to mention your morale, because they'll make you feel exotic, glamorous, and excruciatingly creative!

In my case, I took up jewelry design and bead-making while on leave after Mikey was born. By the time I returned to work, some of that wearable art was of my own creation. Like a huge, nuggetty "faux turquoise" polymer clay necklace I'd made because I didn't want to have to cough up the money for the real thing. It hung almost to my waistline. A real eye-grabber of a statement piece. When I got back, and had to go cover the Grammys, I wore it with the same flowing black tunic and trousers that I practically lived in while I was pregnant. And it worked beautifully. The tunic concealed my middle, which was still some ways from normalcy, and the only thing anyone really noticed was the necklace.

Realize, of course, that the best "cosmetic enhancement" you could use right now is internal. There is NO WAY you can completely disguise that huge stomach. So don't drive yourself crazy trying to do so. You're going to run into so many people who are so much thinner than even the non-pregnant you would ever be.

I remember trying to figure out how to dress strategically and fashionably enough to feel comfortable at an interview with Mick Jagger. I finally settled on my best sartorial friend, the old reliable flowing black fabric top, with hot pink pajama-type trousers underneath, and a long, hot pink chiffon scarf giving me a nice vertical line down the front. Fairly chic, even while extremely front-loaded. Well, it turns out, no one gave a hoot. First, everyone in the room was so much more focused on Mick Jagger

— the man, his music, his film career, and his daughter Jade making him a grandfather. And besides, no one cared after we all noticed the little diamond he had some dentist set into one of his front teeth.

Post-pregnancy plumage, however, will be among the least of your planning concerns for your return to work after maternity leave. There's the critically-important issue of baby-care when you're not there — who, where, how long and how much. And what if you'd rather have it the other way around, at least in spurts?

How does your office manager feel about bringing a baby in from time to time? Does your company have, or might it be leaning toward, a day care center on the premises? Working parents on the Paramount Pictures lot can take advantage of the studio's own day care center, smack dab in the center of the premises. Would your company be open to starting one if you broached the subject? After all, something that benefits not just one employee but many others at the office, might actually be worth consideration.

She went out on maternity leave and then returned, with a crib-away-from-crib in tow.

My first on-air job was at a radio station where the boss's wife was an executive there in her own right. She went out on maternity leave and then returned, with a crib-away-from-crib in tow. It worked wonderfully for her (and later for all of us), to have her infant so close at all times. Fortunately, she was professional and organized enough to handle it along with her job. The only problem was that she shared an office with a male program director, who wasn't crazy about having to work out of a nursery. Nevertheless, he was able to remain a gentleman about it. But they're not all like him!

If you've got your own office space, you'll find much of this easier to manage. Virtually every actress I've covered who's also a mom, Meg Ryan, Demi Moore, and many more, hold enough sway to be able to bring their babies and/or children with them on any of their movie sets. They have entire entourages devoted to the care and support of their little ones while they're filming. Sometimes a whole separate trailer is set aside for a nursery, playroom, or even school. In Rachel Hunter's case, they even take the tutor along when husband Rod Stewart goes out on tour.

The rest of us don't have that luxury. And for that reason, it's an issue you're going to have to think through, and plan for. And sometimes, even if you do have your own office, you run the risk of stepping on toes.

After all, let's not forget what Lynn Redgrave went through years ago, when she wanted to breast feed her baby on the set of *House Calls*. After events on the show failed to resolve to her satisfaction, she wound up working with more lawyers than actors. Needless to say, MANY more aches and pains than she ever had while pregnant or nursing!

There can be drawbacks to bringing the baby to work: You remind everyone of your divided loyalties and your "Mommy track."

I can recall the case of one local TV anchor who was successful enough to earn an add-on to her office so her new baby could have a small nursery. She could return to work sooner, bring her infant with her, have the baby close by to nurse, change, and even play with. A dream come true, right? Well, not to one of her colleagues, a well-established and successful reporter who summarily lost an office for the sake of the anchorwoman's nursery-conversion. Unfortunately, that gave birth to a growing family of inter-office grumblings and vibes that soured toward her.

And there can be drawbacks to bringing the baby to work: You remind everyone of your divided loyalties and your "Mommy track." Furthermore, the arrival of a baby, even for just a few minutes, will mean work stoppage for many of your office mates. Women, and some men, too, will HAVE to come over and take a look. Or they'll want to hold the baby and say coochie-coo. The boss may not appreciate the interruption, unless he or she is also a parent or just very mellow about these things.

How far away from your workplace do you live? How quickly could you get home — either for a baby-fix or a breast feeding session? There's a big one right there, so to speak! More like a couple of them, actually. Breast feeding and the working woman. If you think you can pull off bringing the baby to the office every so often, and you don't have your own office with a door where you can close yourself in, check out the women's lounge. Often women's bathrooms are bigger than men's. You can breast feed, etc. there with at least some privacy.

There's another approach that, in effect, turns your office kitchen's refrigerator into a breast feeder's co-conspirator. Remember, you will HAVE to relieve yourself of that breast milk. It will be rather urgent at times. I used to wake up in the morning feeling as if my breasts were filled with gravel. It was breast milk, inflating me as hard as a couple of cannonballs. And it hurt! There's only one effective solution: find the baby, but fast, and get him or her started siphoning, ASAP.

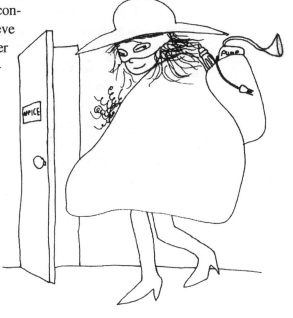

If you're at the office and the baby is not, you'll need to strike up an acquaintance with a breast pump. They're available at most of the better-equipped drug stores, and they're small enough to pack into a large purse or tote bag. You can hide away with it during the average coffee break, take the pressure off, store what you pumped out in the fridge discreetly until you take it home, or throw it out. If it has to be dumped, don't worry. As long as you keep at it, you'll make more.

If you'd rather stash it until you leave for the day and take it home with you, you absolutely MUST label the container, or the bag it's in, with your name on it. After all, almost every office has a refrigerator raider. Or some hapless soul will wind up wondering what was in that coffee creamer they grabbed in a hurry! You must remember to take it home each day, and that it is very perishable. If it's not kept cool — maybe in a cooler bag you'd usually pack a lunch in — it's no good.

While you're planning ahead for all this, expect to stash a box of disposable breast pads in your desk drawer. Because you'll leak! Maybe a lot. And everyone *is* going to know if you don't take precautions.

And since we're really getting personal, include with the breast pads some extra panti-liners. It's not just your middle that will be stretched out of shape for awhile afterwards. There will be lots of exercises recommended for you to do to snap back, some of them rather intimate ones. Do not take these recommendations lying down, so to speak!

As you gear up for all this, try not to dismiss the needs of that other inside of you: your head — not your stomach. You're likely to feel rather self-conscious, and perhaps even a little guilty, as you get bigger. You may find yourself wondering what your coworkers think of you. Do they see you as someone not as committed to the cause anymore? Do you sense some resentment because you have to take a few more or longer breaks, or you "tie up" the lady's room, or it seems as if you're always running off to the doctor? Any jealousy of the attention you're now getting, or the nice long "break" they know you're on the brink of? (If only they knew!)

Is your impending departure adding to their workloads? After all, in some offices, they may not have the budget or the inclination to replace you, and others will be forced to pick up the slack. There may, indeed, be a whiff or two of such discontent.

It might also be more than just a whiff. You may actually lose a friend or two, or eight, in the process. Maybe even some you've been close to for years, who turn unsympathetic when they find that you're no longer shoulder-to-shoulder together on the career-devotion track. I was totally unprepared for this one. I can still recall the jolt I felt when I was told — "I realize you don't give a 'hoot' about MY life anymore!" Frankly, it was an even greater seismic jolt within me to realize that this speaker might be onto something.

You know what? That's exactly how it's supposed to be in your world as it's now turned. Hopefully, those who may no longer seem so friendly will have their own significant-other with more reliable emotional ties than you can offer. If so, remind yourself of that. Your new arrival is the one who comes first from here on.

Try to be as patient as you can, take the high road, by all means hold your tongue! It won't help to start an argument and you're not about to convert anyone. Keep it to yourself. Go ahead and stew about it now, because later on, believe me, you won't have time to worry about it. Years ago, I had some pretty perplexing feelings of my own to suppress, around fellow workaholics who suddenly had a life I didn't relate to after the stork arrived. My focus had been "all career all the time," and I couldn't imagine how it could ever be otherwise. It wasn't until I had a baby of my own that I finally understood.

Still, don't be tempted to turn yourself into a non-stop commercial for your new arrival. A little goes a very long way, particularly at your workplace. Once I made the mistake of whipping out a brand new picture of an ultrasound of my budding Elizabeth. I was almost knocked over by the weight of the eyeballs rolling and hands smacking into foreheads around the assignment desk. All that is best left at home with family members and really close friends who truly will appreciate it. Some people find it boring when coworkers chatter endlessly about their little Poopsie.

There's one critical thing to keep in mind here; for your sanity's sake, even as you still aim to be a kind and cooperative team player to the bitter end (with the raging emotional and hormonal hurricanes that accompany the construction job going on behind your bellybutton): THEY'LL THINK WHAT THEY'RE GOING TO THINK — NO MATTER WHAT YOU DO!

AND YOU CAN'T HELP THAT! SO STOP WORRYING ABOUT IT!

Don't make all the conflicting opinions around you more important than they should be. It doesn't really matter in the greater scheme of things. It's what they may not realize that IS important. Which, in the long run, is that you are now onto bigger and better things for your own life. Remember this if anyone in the office makes like they want to give you a complex — as some competitive and resolutely single souls out there may be tempted to do. It will help you maintain balance and perspective.

It's wise to keep ALL these ruminations STRICTLY to yourself. As you readjust your inner view-finder, don't confide the gory details to anyone, especially those you work with. Regardless of how close a friendship has been, there is no guarantee that it'll stay that way, now that your co-workers no longer have all your attention to themselves. Even if you're positive they understand exactly where you're coming from, they don't need your brutal honesty. Feelings you thought you were so sure about will be knocked WAY out of whack if you even suggest that some concern of theirs has now plummeted a few hundred miles on your priority scale. This much frankness will likely mark the beginning of the end of those friendships.

Don't make all the conflicting opinions around you more important than they should be. It doesn't really matter in the greater scheme of things.

Your social scene around work and beyond will sort itself out in any event, as connections unravel with some childless friends and colleagues, and tighten with others who share the parenthood bond. Just know this: as fabulous as the job (or anyone attached to it) may be, it doesn't — and can never — love you back. On the other hand the little person you mother always will.

Tips 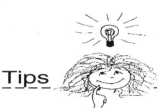 To Remember

✓ You'll have to run for cover when you're pregnant — whether it involves what you're wearing, who you're toting, or how you're feeling.

✓ Know your own needs, stresses, job demands, activity levels, and expanding size when you choose maternity clothes. Nice things can be found in maternity shops, but sometimes the better stuff is in your closet already. Some maternity shops still don't get it right, and won't have appropriate or professional-looking clothes to offer.

✓ Stick to single colors, easy fit, and anything that emphasizes the vertical rather than the horizontal. Comfortable (and most likely flat) shoes are essential. Investigate ethnic, hand-crafted and one-of-a-kind garments that cover you nicely and add a little panache! They might even be cheaper, and lovely enough to continue enjoying after your figure returns. Which may take longer than expected.

✓ Examine your options once baby is here. Is it possible to bring him or her to work with you?

✓ Does the office have a day care center for employees' kids? Do you have your own office space that can accommodate your little one? Can you even bring the baby in for a visit — or would they frown on such things?

✓ Do you have a place to breastfeed while at work? Consider bringing a breast pump in if you can't bring the baby. Will you need to store the breastmilk for later use, or just toss it? Or, do you live near enough where you can "bug out" for a nursing break?

✓   Will your coworkers be annoyed by any of this? Or feel put out? Or even betrayed because your baby now comes before everyone and everything else? Prepare for your shifted priorities to knock someone's nose out of joint, and compromise a friendship. Even long-running friendships can be vulnerable.

✓   You must try to be gracious, NOT obnoxious about your baby, nor hostile toward others who may be in conflict with you.

✓   And be discreet about your feelings! There's no need to offend anyone by your new single-mindedness.

✓   Your social situation will sort itself out, and you'll appreciate the unconditional love of your little one even more.

Chapter 4

The Assistance League

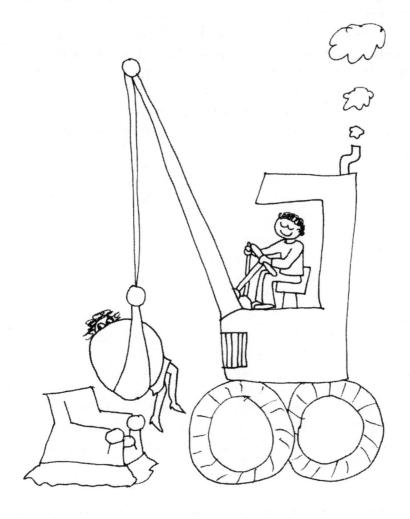

HE'S got to help. He helped get you into this, didn't he? I'm happy to report that it's a rare man who shies away from attending his baby's birth. And thank goodness, too, because he should witness, not only the wonders of the two of you becoming three, but the strain and pain it puts you through. At least he should be momentarily "floored," and even more in awe of you.

Involving your spouse from the beginning will help you toward a united front on "Planet Baby." Bring him in with you on as many obstetrician appointments as you can. Let him hear the early heartbeat and watch the ultrasound. Don't hold off until Lamaze class. Encourage him to be masseur and chef (read: *Associate Baby Builder*) and big-ticket operator — like assembling the crib or other put-to-gethers, moving the baby furniture around in the nursery, or even painting the walls. As you enter the home stretch, have him take therapeutic walks with you. It will help him prepare to be your coach in the delivery room.

Involving your spouse from the beginning will help you toward a united front on "Planet Baby."

As Elizabeth's arrival date loomed, I made more and more use of Bruce. He sanded and painted furniture for the baby room, then assembled it and moved it into place. Bruce had to do everything from hoisting me out of chairs and beds to tying my sneaker laces, which I could no longer SEE, let alone reach. He shuttled me to and from work assignments, especially at night. He barbecued endless platters of turkey legs for me. He nagged me into going on low-impact hikes and treadmill trips with him. He counted out my pregnancy vitamins for me each day. He was great!

Another thing he did which may sound silly, but felt great, was to pull me around in the neighborhood swimming pool. By the end of my pregnancy, the water's anti-gravity effect greatly relieved my anguished back and swollen legs and ankles. Since I could hardly move, no less do exercises, Bruce would walk around the pool with a long rope, literally towing me through the water. (This worked wonders for my morale.)

And yes, I did say morale. Even at the pool. While I was prodigiously pregnant. And nothing but wasp-like waistlines between the tiniest slivers of bikinis had stationed themselves in plain sight at all 360 degrees around the pool. Every last one studded with the loveliest and most diminutive of bellybuttons. At this late date, my stomach was so distended that I'd gone past having one anymore. What was left of my bellybutton had begun to "blow OUT" the other way! Seeing to the bottom of your belly button can really be startling. Until times like this, it never really occurs to you that there IS 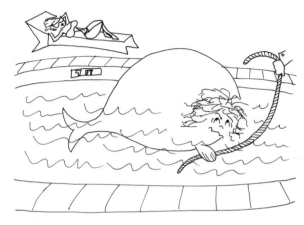 a bottom to it. Impossible enough, Bruce still had eyes only for me.

As you count down the last days wondering when it's all gonna be over with, there's a lot you can do to keep from losing your mind over all the suspense. (It'll greatly depend on how you feel.)

One approach is to get really busy. I mean REALLY busy. You can use the distraction to ease your nervousness. Book up your time as much as you can stand, and work in all those lunches and/or shopping trips with the friends you probably won't see too much of after the baby comes. Go visiting. Finish all those baby shower thank-you notes. If your husband can get away for a midday break with you, so much the better. At night, hit the restaurants (the nice grown-up ones), the movies, dinner theaters, or go catch some live music somewhere together. Later on, you WON'T have much time or energy for activities like these. And even if you DO have the time and energy, you may not be able to find a good baby-sitter.

Another approach, is what to do if you're too huge to want to move. You may be too tired, swollen, achy, and grumpy to do much of anything, let alone go out. In that case, use this time to rest. Keep a journal about your life and feelings right now.

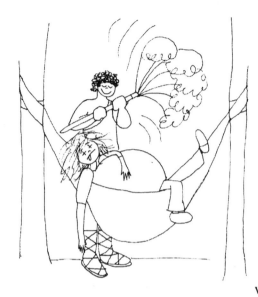

Be kind and indulgent to yourself, and enjoy each other in the peace and quiet you'll soon be kissing good-bye. It'll be the last time, for a LOOOOONNNNNGGGGG time, that there will be just the two of you.

If you have an eagerly helpful man around, doting on you, realize that what you also have is your own personal, always-on-call masseur. Bruce was as good to me as Warren Beatty in that department. Maybe better, for all I know. When the movie *Bugsy* was being promoted, and Beatty's impending parenthood with Annette Bening was the big Hollywood buzz, he thought nothing of leaving a group of reporters waiting so he could stroll over to where she was — with her own group of reporters. Soon enough, his hands would be all over the back of her neck and shoulders, working seriously on each little muscle knot before she began taking questions. When I went home that night, my own version of Warren Beatty went on duty again, working on the muscle knots all over the back of MY neck and shoulders.

Confidentially speaking, by all means consult your doctor about further intimacy together even at this time. You may not be able to perform too much, but there are still lots of pleasures to be had. And since he has the more flexible mid-section right now, let him do the work!

One really neat way to enjoy each other is to have your picture taken together, while you're this big. It may seem a little corny when you do, but years later, you'll look back on those photos with warmth and wonder, and awe at how you ballooned! I wanted a few such snapshots to keep people from talking. One interview I did in the latter stages of pregnancy was with one of my longtime heroes, Mel Brooks. When I asked if I could have my picture taken with him, he more than agreed. I didn't realize 'til after the Polaroid image came in that he'd puffed out his chest, smiled REEEEEEEEEEEEALLY wide, and with one arm around my shoulders, his other hand was showing off my belly with a gesture of bigtime pride. (My one and only opportunity to feel like Anne Bancroft, I guess.)

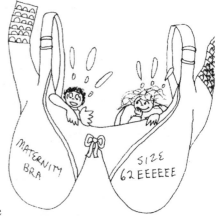

You may even want your husband to take a private snapshot of you, in the altogether, for you to amaze yourself with, after your waistline's come back. I particularly enjoyed pretending I was Demi Moore on the cover of *Vanity Fair*. And I had Bruce take an extra Polaroid of me from the chest up. I knew I would never be this Dolly-Parton-esque again, and I wanted to make sure I had evidence of it. (I had enough to be Dolly Parton's mother.) I know some women who were so fanatical that they had pictures taken of themselves at regular intervals through the pregnancy. What they wound up with was a kind of flip book of a ripening fruit. This little side adventure is one you'll both appreciate, now AND later.

Also, don't neglect whatever photos you may have from any ultrasound procedures. We even have copies of the chromosome counts of each of our kids, because I was considered old enough to need extensive genetic testing both times.

You'll need your mate to be your coach in the maternity ward. Direct him to pack your hospital bag for you, let him throw in a few things of his own invention that he thinks you'd like, and have him carry it all in for you. Bruce rather liked the bribery approach. He stuck a handful of imported chocolate bars into my hospital bag, and passed them out to every obstetrical nurse on the floor. They were very attentive around my labor room. (I'm sure they would have been, anyway.) AND, they bestowed the "World Class Coach" award upon him by the time it was over (which he deserved, chocolate bars or not).

I'm still impressed about the things he took care of behind the scenes while I was preoccupied with my babies' "coming out parties." He even contributed a couple of pairs of his socks to my hospital kit. Those (and the robe I forgot that HE remembered to pack for me) came in handy while he was parking the car and unpacking my suitcase, and I was sent to the hallways to walk. And walk. And walk some more, as the contractions started to get serious.

Unfortunately, that made him miss one of the big chuckles leading up to Mikey's birth. My Long Walk through the maternity ward halls before my son's delivery occurred exactly one night after *Murphy Brown* had delivered her baby boy on TV. (You know, the one Dan Quayle once got some political mileage out of.) I'll never forget the middle-aged couple, no doubt visiting some new mom they loved, strolling past me and murmuring — "Look! 'Murphy Brown!'" The one time in my life I looked like Candice Bergen! It must have been the bathrobe and socks.

You're apt to want the birth "documented," so let your mate make the arrangements to videotape the birth or take pictures. He may decide to recruit a mutual friend, although you can hire professionals also. Or, he may feel so indispensable and all-powerful by then that he wants to do it himself.

By the way, if it sounds weird to think of having somebody ELSE in there with you, looking on, especially THERE, while you're in active labor, don't let it bother you too much. By the time you're deeply into it, you won't care if the Cavalry thunders through. Trust me, you'll be just a little TOO BUSY!! My mother came marching in at the exact moment Mikey was emerging, and I was in the most awkward and compromising of positions, and that didn't phase me, either. I was "in conference," as it were. Let your man oversee all this, anyway. It'll give him something else to feel important about. You've got other things to do.

After Elizabeth arrived, Bruce smuggled the biggest, baddest, sloppiest double cheeseburgers into the hospital for me every day. AND diet sodas, which I'd given up for the duration and was now craving like mad. HE wanted to be the one to change the baby for the first time, which was fine by me. And this time, I took the pictures. Don't pass this one up, by the way. Believe me, you WILL get equal time! And if your man is hesitant about such things, cheer him on by telling him that even Chuck Norris himself couldn't measure up with such valor. For all his black belt skills and courage, and the multitudes of bad guys and bad situations he's overcome, Norris admitted to me during an interview that the thought of confronting his baby's used diapers made him want to go hide somewhere.

If you're the least bit picky about schools, the same ones you'll like best are the ones that everyone else likes best.

It'll be your man's job to outfit the car with the correct and legal baby-seat the hospital will insist you have before you can leave. And, for the first few days at home, when you're supposed to be physically inert, he will be and should be doing all the driving.

Something else HE can handle for you while you're recovering, involves some of the long-range planning you'll both be busy with in the years ahead. What kind of bank accounts do you want to set up, for example? Let him deal with the banks, the accountants, the brokers, the IRS, the markets, the options, the research, all the other whatevers and, of course, all the forms!

And that's not all.

Far too many new moms, and dads, too, find out too late, and with eyeballs rolling back up into their heads in great dismay, that they've missed a deadline in their little one's future. Preschool, for example, what virtually no one thinks to tell you early-on is that if you're the least bit picky about schools, the ones you'll like best are the same ones that everyone else likes best. Therefore, you'll have to get your name on a waiting list, but fast!

It's always been a little perplexing to me that anyone would even have to think about something like this when the baby's so young! I mean, isn't this pushing things a little? Certainly yes, but frankly, no. The most popular schools will likely start taking names after the baby's born. (They won't let you sign on while you're still pregnant.) They'll all tell you, quite honestly, that the sooner you get your name on their list, the greater opportunity you'll have three years later when it's time for school to start. This is research your husband can help you with. You'll eventually have to decide whether you want two, three, or five-days-a-week classes, mornings only, afternoons only, and so forth, plus how you'll budget for those. And your husband can be the one to register your child in the school.

Not only did Bruce prepare the nursery for us both, but he was constantly delivering me water refills once Elizabeth and I had moved in. If you breast feed, you'll be thirstier than ever. I really made Bruce work. I even sent him to get this industrial-strength breast cream at the drug store after Mikey had been with us a little while. Mikey was so eager to eat that he wore grooves into the sides of me, and I had to resort to some external pain relief.

When Elizabeth came home and settled in, Bruce hovered close and did our bidding as she and I took to our bed, together, and let the rest of the world go on without us. For a couple of weeks I lived that way. You may feel the deepest, almost bestial, mother-wolf or mother-tiger feelings stirring, that makes you want to retire to the back of the cave with your new cub and growl at interlopers. I felt that way with both Elizabeth and Mikey when I burrowed in deeply with each of them. Plus by the time Mikey was here, Elizabeth needed looking after and even with a nanny (whom we had for awhile) she loved, she felt needy of parental affections. So it was often Daddy to the rescue while Mommy was preoccupied with little Brother.

Conveniently enough, both Elizabeth and Mikey were happy to sleep on my chest, and for the first three weeks or so, were light-weight enough to be comfortable for me. You'll come to marvel at the time-table Mother Nature seems to have built in — that the baby doesn't start coming to life and wiggling a lot until somewhere into the second week — about the same time that YOU feel up to coming to life and wiggling a lot. In the meantime, someone still needs to get up and answer the phone, run to the store at an odd hour, or do another load of laundry (and beware: you're in for THOUSANDS of these). Which is where your husband can be a godsend.

Simply remind yourselves that this is on-the-job-training, because you're just beginning to get a feel of the task that's ahead for the two of you. From those late-night feeding relay races and arguments you always hear about — onward. You need to work as a team now. Remember that this is a joint-production that demands an astounding amount of energy, emotion, and waking-hours — and that's just up to now.

You'll both be sleep-deprived, BIG TIME, which means grumpy. YOU, in particular, will be in the throes of postpartum mood swings. Don't EVER underestimate these. Try to keep a grip, even when you think you're already COPING. Your mate, under stresses of his own (which your mood swings will, uh, shall we say — embellish), will be touchy, too.

And then there's the little one, who when in a fit of colic, can work up one heck of a mountainous lather. A colicky baby really does nothing but fuss and cry, at times for hours on end. Apparently for no reason. You'll both be feeling like you're on the ropes trying to figure out how to make your little one more content. And you'll need each other a LOT when this happens (at three in the morning, more often than not).

YOU, in particular, will be in the throes of postpartum mood swings. Don't EVER underestimate these.

Early on, one of the colic depths I hit with Elizabeth lasted for an entire day, beginning in the wee hours when I tried to get her to stop crying. I hugged. I kissed. I checked and rechecked her diapers. I rocked. I carried. I went for drives and strolls around the neighborhood. I fed. I cuddled. I nursed. I provided rides on top of the dryer (the warmth, purring, and regular vibrations of the machine sometimes work very nicely). At the end of this dismaying day, I threw up my hands. Then I racked my brain for the eighteen-dozenth time and realized I'd thought of everything. I was out of ideas beyond carrying her to her crib, setting the lights and the music low, walking away, and shutting the door behind me.

Bruce took partnership that night to a high point. He made me a nice cup of tea, his encouragement and approval of my solution was heartwarming and then made me a fire in the fireplace so I could sit and "decompress." When we checked back on Elizabeth about a half-hour later, she was fast asleep.

It's a great idea to have your mate check into the parental leave policies where HE works. They might have some in effect for new fathers. If they don't, suggest he start some there. If they do, exploit them for all they're worth! You'll BOTH need it. Especially since it takes both you and the baby about two to three weeks, physically, to come back up for air, and reinforcements will be absolutely essential. For all you know, your husband might decide to investigate a work-at-home arrangement for himself. He'll be mighty glad he did, and so will you.

Feed and nurture his creativity whenever you can, as you both start to get the hang of it. Sometimes the Y-chromosomes have impressive ideas to contribute. One of Elizabeth's early colicky nights was solved when Bruce decided Elizabeth should be bundled in a fluffy, warm towel for a few moments. Maybe to remind her of where she'd just recently come from. So a towel was put in the dryer, then taken out and cooled off. Then we wrapped her up in it. To our amazement, her crying stopped stone cold. Her eyes grew big and round as she stared at us, as though she instinctively realized that something important had happened. We laid her down on our bed and observed her closely. She immediately relaxed. Wet her diapers, and fell asleep. And my boy Brucie thought this up. How 'bout that?

Having your husband take an active role at baby time is like seed money — you'll never dream how well it can pay off. Since he can't birth it himself, this is a way he can feel like a prominent part of it. As the baby grows, and you re-establish yourself on the job, he'll be used to pitching in. Let them both conk out together for a catnap in the middle of the afternoon. To encourage physical bonding between father and child that is very beneficial.

Is he curious about your breast milk while you're nursing? Oh, go on, give him some, too! You'd be stunned to know how many new parents share this little secret.

And it goes without saying how many intimate fringe benefits THAT little exchange can provoke! I can't stress this enough. The more you can do, as early as possible, to involve the father in the birth process, the better for mother, father, and child!

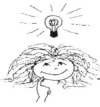

Tips To Remember

✓ Your spousal unit need not feel left out of things, simply because HE'S not having the baby! Making your pregnancy and delivery a TRULY joint production will be great for both of you!

✓ Find out if he's eligible for parental leave from work. Or if he could help initiate such a program if there are none where he works.

✓ Your mate's participation goes WAY beyond Lamaze class. He can be involved in your exercise or health programs, your meal preparation, the nursery preparation, errand-running, phone answering, home management, helping you get out of bed and dress, and planning campaigns of all kinds (from financial to schooling).

✓ He can assist, whichever way you decide to spend your last days of pregnancy — either activity-filled, or just resting up. Now is the time to squeeze in your last few just-the-two-of-you dates before you permanently become a threesome.

✓ Take pictures of you, or you both, and your expanding stomach. Keep a journal.

✓ Encourage his creativity, whether it's packing you up for the hospital, or dealing with a colicky baby later on.

✓ And certainly let him try as much diaper-changing as he wants.

✓ Make sure he has his own bonding time with the baby.

✓ Offer him a once-in-a-lifetime bonding chance with you. Let him taste your breast milk.

✓ Expect the strange new stresses and challenges to get to BOTH of you. Same thing for sleep deprivation. And yes, expect to have arguments. Sometimes at very late hours!

✓ The more he's involved now, the more he'll be used to pitching in later.

Chapter 5
They NEVER Warn You About THIS One!

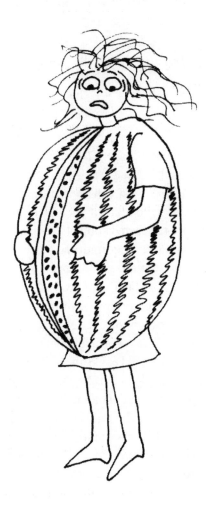

Exactly how close are you to Planet Baby? Still orbiting, or is the landing sequence about to get underway? If so, I'm about to give you some of the best advice I wished I'd had and didn't know about until it was too late. I was given only a mere glancing hint of it when I interviewed Cindy Williams of "Laverne and Shirley" fame with just a few months to go before Elizabeth's arrival. After the interview was over, she pulled me aside, looked me straight in the belly, and warned me about the rigors ahead on delivery day. I'll never forget it — she said "it's like pooping a watermelon." And I'll also never forget how little I grasped the full significance of that.

It felt as if an elf had crawled up inside of me with a baseball bat, and had beaten me up in there.

Don't you make that same mistake. The following is something you should consider, seriously, if you, too, are still waiting to deliver. Certainly, NO ONE thought to offer THIS little recommendation to me. And considering these times, I'll admit it may be a bit controversial. But it helped me profoundly, and I have never once hesitated to pass it on.

The inspiration for this occurred about 4:30 in the morning, after Elizabeth's birth at 10:25 the previous night. The epidural I had during childbirth was all but a memory. A most unfortunate thing. I'd dozed off once I'd been taken back to my room, and awoke a few hours later in the worst pain I'd ever experienced in my life. It felt as if an elf had crawled up inside of me with a baseball bat, and had beaten me up in there. It hurt so much that I cried. Sobbed, actually.

I called for the nurse. She arrived in a few minutes. It felt like much longer, of course. She looked at my chart, and looked at me, then offered me what was on the chart. Tylenol with codeine. I accepted. And I waited. And kept waiting. And nothing happened.

If anything, the pain got worse. I called her again. She returned, and offered me a hemorrhoid pad. Nothing topical would come close to addressing THIS kind of pain. She said there was nothing else she could give me and she refused to call the doctor in the dead of night for a stronger prescription. I remained in agony for several more hours until she deemed it proper to call the doctor without waking anyone up unnecessarily.

A stronger remedy was prescribed and given to me, and only at that point did the pain subside.

What was it? A total of three shots of morphine through that day. I was in a stupor, but what did I care? The baby was sleeping on my shoulder, and I hardly moved. Whatever the baby needed (which wasn't much) the nurses were coming in to check upon at frequent intervals. Mostly, she slept like a log. My milk hadn't come in yet, so there wasn't any breast feeding to do, or to offer. And she didn't seem to want any. We both dozed the day away together. And the pain subsided.

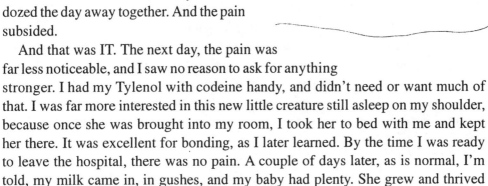

And that was IT. The next day, the pain was far less noticeable, and I saw no reason to ask for anything stronger. I had my Tylenol with codeine handy, and didn't need or want much of that. I was far more interested in this new little creature still asleep on my shoulder, because once she was brought into my room, I took her to bed with me and kept her there. It was excellent for bonding, as I later learned. By the time I was ready to leave the hospital, there was no pain. A couple of days later, as is normal, I'm told, my milk came in, in gushes, and my baby had plenty. She grew and thrived both mentally and physically, and is still doing so to this day.

This is a long, roundabout way of addressing the touchy subject of medications and the brand new mom. How do you feel about drugs for pain, during and/or after delivery? Are you one of those stalwart souls determined to do it all naturally? If you ARE inclined to go it au naturelle, I salute you with 21 guns blazing. I'm not made of stuff that strong. I wasn't in that delivery room to earn a medal of valor, or even a diamond of any size! So I remained open to whatever might be needed.

Epidural? You bet! And yes, an epidural is something to swear by. Some women I know tell of being out in public, very pregnant, when a total stranger whisks by and whispers "epidural" for no reason. Well, we who've delivered KNOW the reason! It alleviates the PAIN! It isn't completely pain-free, in and of itself, though. Know, going in, that the installation of the epidural will be the cause of some discomfort. Sometimes gaspingly so when the anesthesiologist actually inserts it in your back. And it also means you're going to be hooked up to an IV. They go hand-in-hand. There are moments when I think back on all this and remember THAT as one of the roughest parts to suffer through.

But what about the hours AFTER the main event, when the epidural has long since faded? No one seems to think that far ahead, at least about this. So let me do the honors. The most urgent problem to deal with, the first day or so after delivery is pain that might be substantial. It could hurt longer if you deliver by cesarean. Know this: IF IT IS NOT WRITTEN ON YOUR CHART, IN BLACK AND WHITE, AND IN ADVANCE, you will NOT get it.

And at 4:30 in the morning, you may not be able to get ANYTHING written into your chart. Studies have shown that doctors routinely err on the conservative side, and

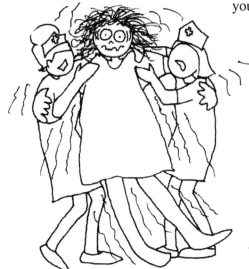

under-prescribe medication in many circumstances. Speak to your own doctor about this beforehand, maybe at about the sixth or seventh month while you still have plenty of time to wrap up loose ends. Get everything agreed to, and in writing, IN ADVANCE, that IF you need a narcotic for pain relief after delivery, one is already prescribed for you.

As I discovered, it did NOT ruin my life. It did not turn me, or my daughter, into hopeless junkies. It was not evidence of some deep character flaw within me. It did not impact my milk supply. I needed it for exactly one day, and haven't wanted it since. I do not, repeat, do NOT advocate heavy drug use. Heaven knows, when you're establishing yourself on Planet Baby you need ALL your wits about you. But I never forgot this — pardon the expression — painful lesson.

When I was pregnant with Mikey, I discussed this with my doctor, and arranged everything in advance. And guess what happened? Maybe it was because this was my second birth and I was, shall we say, broken in. Maybe not. But the next day, the pain wasn't anywhere near as severe as it was after Elizabeth was born. This time, I didn't even bother with that prescription, but I'm glad it was available just in case. I'd have HATED to be without it.

There are a couple of other matters deserving of fair warnings well in advance, that you're also not apt to hear much about. And I'm very happy I lived through both to tell the tale.

Right after delivery, you may find that your body has decided to take the rest of the day off. Or at least go WAY out to lunch. You're in for this ESPECIALLY if you've just been through something drastic, from an epidural to a cesarean. It will seem as though your nether regions decided to stay numbed out. You will be unable to go to the bathroom effectively beyond urinating. You may go through two or three days, eating quite well, and beginning to feel — uh, shall we say — backed up, knowing it's got to come out the other end sooner or later. And not only will you be temporarily unable to (since that part of you has momentarily stopped working because of the anesthesia), you'll be terrified to try. You'll be afraid that you'll rip yourself open again in the very area already ripped up pretty radically from your baby's delivery.

> *Right after delivery, you may find that your body has decided to take the rest of the day off. Or at least go WAY out to lunch.*

Try not to let it panic you! This is normal! It's supposed to work this way. Your fears will pass, as will whatever non-digestibles need to find their way to the exit. By the time the second or third day has gone by, you won't care if it hurts, anyway. You'll just need to go, and your body will decide at about the same time that it's ready to get with the program again. And when you do, you'll wonder what you were so worried about.

Another truly lovely after-birthing trauma is known among us survivors as "the shakes." Within hours of Elizabeth's arrival, the nurses came in to visit me and suggested that I try to go to the bathroom. I agreed. But only my mind got up with one smooth motion and did so. The rest of me began to shake like the San Andreas Fault. My legs, arms, torso, everything from approximately the scalp down felt like it was inside the paint-mixing machine at the hardware store. Thank goodness there were two nurses who'd dropped in. I needed one of them to prop me up on each side. Fortunately, this phenomenon lasted only about as long as that first trip to and from the commode — at least for the physical side of me. And it happened only with my first baby, not my second. But my mind can still get a little unsettled by the thought of it.

Whenever I think back on any of this, memories of a conversation with Mary Steenburgen come to mind. She, too, adores being a mother of two. She also adored the act of BECOMING the mother of two. She told me that if someone said she would be going into labor again, one minute from now, she'd be happier than a clam.

Tips To Remember

✓ Giving birth is what Cindy Williams describes as "pooping a watermelon." Therefore, you can expect it to hurt.

✓ Decide in advance whether your goal is completely natural childbirth or delivery assisted by pain medication.

✓ Many women swear by epidural anesthesia, to get through the roughest part of labor. It alleviates contraction pains but requires the use of an I V and an automatic blood pressure cuff.

✓ You may need a stronger pain reliever AFTER delivery. Perhaps something powerful. Especially if it's your first. And particularly if you've had a cesarean.

✓ You will NOT get a narcotic or other strong medication unless you have your doctor's approval IN ADVANCE.

✓ Discuss this with your doctor IN ADVANCE, and GET IT IN WRITING ON YOUR CHART. You're apt to need it for only a day or so, and won't suffer any harm. Nor will it affect your baby. The effects will wear off well before you're able to breastfeed.

✓ Be prepared for "the shakes," following delivery. Especially if it's your first. Your body will shake and tremble, making it difficult to get out of bed. This condition will pass quickly.

✓ If you've had any anesthesia, be prepared to have some difficulty using the bathroom for the first one to three days. The medication will slow down your system so you may not be able to do more than void your bladder. Don't worry that you'll further strain the birthing area.

✓ Your system will return to normal after all of the above.

Chapter 6
Clothes Calls

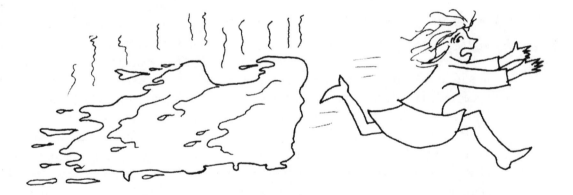

Something finally came between me and my Calvins. Happened every day, in fact, when I'd segue from work chasing celebrities for the AP to my other job (the one at home chasing children). Dressing nicely for work has always been important to me, whether I was a writer, news anchor, talk show host, or entertainment reporter, because I'd need an air of credibility and would have to at least appear as though I'm a little bit "with it." It's the same for most working women. But there are lots of things I love in my closet that I have not worn since I first became pregnant with Elizabeth (who's now seven).

It's not because these garments don't fit me anymore. It's because I like them too much, and have invested too much in them, to get rid of them. Items like suede trousers and skirts. Fine silk blouses. Really high heels. A favorite big-name designer jacket or outfit. I know they'll hold up because I put them away carefully and their design is classic, so they'll still be in "style" in a decade or so. And I'm fully prepared NOT to wear any of these clothes again until both my kids are well out of the peanut-butter-and-goo stage. I've accepted that — and because of Mikey, who's five — I'm realistically looking at another few years. I've had to fight off my vanity and be okay with that.

I'm fully prepared NOT to wear any of these clothes again until both my kids are well out of the peanut-butter-and-goo stage.

If you've got to follow a trend or two, go for accessories like shoes, scarves or jewelry, that don't take up much space in your closet or your budget, and can be changed, tossed aside, or messed with in the wink of some designer's eye. You'll find them in the most unexpected places. A collector's item I picked up with great delight was actually presented to me after an interview with B.B. King. He made it a habit to carry with him a handful of little guitar-shaped pins that he'd give out on a moment's notice. Imagine my pride when he looked me in the eye, and then in the gut, and with a smile said, "and YOU get two!"

Many outdated or worn-out garments can be recycled into dress-up or fairy princess garb for a little girl. Or school and Halloween stuff for a girl OR boy. Practically speaking, you'll want to save your big bucks for other things, instead, like food and laundry supplies in bulk (you'll be astounded at how fast supplies get used up), karate lessons, music camp, braces, bikes, home improvements, or an occasional Mondo Barbie if you simply MUST indulge. In fact, Barbie's very likely to be far better dressed than you'll be for years!

If you have to dress up for work, you must be ready to make "the mad dash" within the first few seconds of coming home at the end of the day. Be prepared for your child to want to greet you right away, and turn you into a climbing tree. Mine basically want me to wear THEM. And, you know something? You'll come to crave this. Which will be fortunate, because for a long time, as they grow and grow and grow, they'll still want you to "uppie" them.

You'll also want to wipe off your makeup, as Ann Jillian pointed out to me, because while they're young, they'll want to nibble on your face. Which her little boy, Andy Joe, did all the time. She wouldn't wear any makeup around the house while she was off-duty.

Train yourself for a moment's reality-check first. You will have to make it a habit to run, not walk, to your bedroom or closet or other safety zone and change out of your work clothes as quickly as possible. You may have someone wanting to crawl up onto your lap the second you sit down. Your child may want not simply to approach you but to tackle you. If you're holding something that could cut, snag, smear or spill, count on that to happen.

I always keep a stack of indestructibles like T-shirts and sweat pants in plain sight and within easy reach whenever I have to make a quick change out of a nice suit. No fumbling through a drawer. You may have some-one trying to ride you at that exact moment.

Whenever my kids approach me, I first scan their faces for goop. They always want to kiss me and bury their faces in my thighs. I'm positive they're trying to find their way back "in." At times like this, you'd better be wearing something invincible. Second, I check their hands. What's on them — and in them. Not only is it important to see that they've been in the mud or the ketchup, but what they're holding that might be pointed at you.

I was about to leave for work early one morning, dressed in a delicious cream-colored outfit, all ready to meet George Clooney, with whom I had an interview scheduled later in the day. An obvious reason to want to look as nice as possible, 'eh? My son gave me a good-bye hug which I eagerly accepted. I didn't realize until I was halfway out the door that he'd had an open, hot-pink, felt-tip marker in his hand, its pointed end aimed directly at my stomach. I wound up with lost time, lost money (gone to dry cleaners), temporarily lost outfit, and briefly and most regrettably, lost temper. I'm just grateful he hadn't picked up a knife, for both our sakes. These things happen awfully fast.

I also found that my defensive scanning reflex had to be expanded very quickly beyond just my little people and myself — outward to most of the furniture, especially anything that even remotely involves food. Better know what you're getting into when you're approaching the dinner table. You may be about to sit down on a puddle of pudding, or a smear of Spaghettios. Or relax into the back of a chair, dining room OR otherwise, that your kid just gummed, or finger-painted with strained cherries, bacon grease, or even old non-edible standards like paint.

When they were little, both my kids regularly found ways to eat their meals with their backs turned to the table, and their faces and hands all over the chair backs. Still do now, at times. Which means I sometimes head off for work in the morning with the image of their most recent cuisine impressed upon the back of my blouse or jacket like some T-shirt slogan. If you haven't spotted it in time, believe me, it will spot you, instead.

I felt bad about this and thought it was just my not being vigilant, until I interviewed Michael McDonald for one of his solo albums. He confessed to me with both embarrassment AND pride about a business meeting he attended while wearing a little dribble of baby barf on the back of his shirt. Seems his little pumpkin had stealthily anointed him JUST after he'd picked the baby up to say good-bye for the day. I tell you, this HAPPENS!

I've worn that kind of souvenir to work with me, too, and more. Sometimes I'll look like the napkin my children SHOULD have used after breakfast. Because I WAS! One time I was busy taking notes at a Bruce Willis news conference for *Die Hard Two* only to realize halfway through that the back of one of my trouser legs was drizzled with droppings from my daughter's favorite dish — strained bananas. How it got on the bottom of my pants when she was eating at table-height I have yet to figure out.

It doesn't even necessarily have to be food. Nose slime will do fine. As will pre-fab items. Like the troll stickers on my pants legs which I noticed after arriving at Disneyland — to cover Elizabeth Taylor's 60th birthday bash. I was just climbing out of my car, ready to trundle over to where reporters were gathering for the tram-ride to the press area, when MY Elizabeth took over all my concentration. My trouser hems were studded with the shiny little troll stickers that my daughter was decorating everything in sight with before I left on assignment. At least with those, you can quickly get rid of the evidence, and hopefully without too many witnesses.

The best kid-friendly wear is anything that's okay to mistreat. Because mistreated it will be. That means stained, snagged, unraveled, stretched out of shape, ripped, and snipped — just wait 'til the young 'un discovers the Wonderful World of Scissors for the very first time! Not only that, but it also better be washing machine-friendly, because that's where it's likely to spend the most time.

Clothes Calls

And dare we say, where you, too, will be spending a lot of time. I've been at this for some years now, and I'm still impressed by the amount of laundry we generate in one day. Some days you'll feel as though you opened up a laundry business. And as with your heart on your sleeve, you'll wear the results, if you're not on constant alert.

You may find you have to plan laundry affairs as carefully as you plan a staff meeting. To keep track of who needs what on how soon a morning. For us it's — "is she at Brownies tomorrow (for which she needs her Brownie uniform washed), or is it the full dress uniform? Can I squeeze two loads in before I drop, including his karate gi for tomorrow afternoon, that I won't be around to wash in the morning?" Oh yes, and can I get the chocolate ice cream stain out of it? Will my husband be upset when he sees all those pink boxer shorts in his underwear drawer (because I was running late and accidentally threw everything together with a new red kid's T-shirt)? And that old urban legend about missing socks? Just wait 'til you add a whole bunch of little socks to that equation!

By the way, I have a suggestion for that one. Check the back of the blouse you've put on, before you leave in the morning. One of those AWOL socks just might be stuck to it. I went through a couple of hours in the studio sweating over a hot tape deck without realizing I'd been wearing a little white lace-cuffed sock on my back, thanks to the fabled static cling from the dryer. Your husband is also a VERY easy target for this. You may find you need to do one load of big stuff, towels and grown-up clothes, and one safely isolated load for all the teensy kid stuff.

There will be many times when you won't be able to change out of your good clothes in a hurry. Or when you want to, or have to, take the little one out with you and you'd rather not look like a condemned building with legs. Here, too, please! Nothing that will shrivel up and die if your kid's plate of spaghetti decides to drop in!

Darker colors are always preferable — not to mention slimming! Black is best. Yeah, okay, it can be drab. Maybe *Vogue* magazine doesn't like it this season. But that's where all those lovely and versatile accessories come in, right? What you'll appreciate most is that it won't show stains, dirt, or finger marks — at least not as obviously as something lighter-colored would. You'll be able to find plenty of accessories to go with it. And heaven forbid, you might actually look somewhat fashionable. You can always opt for brown or navy if you prefer. You may wish to borrow a scheme that Jackie Onassis was said to have used — within your own means, of course. If you find something really fabulous and work-able, buy several. In the same color and others, too. If your munchkin sends it permanently to the Land of Oz, simply don the duplicate and everybody stays happy — even you.

I also liked elasticized waistlines. Still do, I'm afraid. They're much more forgiving if you're edging back into conventional clothes after pregnancy and need size options for awhile. High heels, for all their allure, can be a problem when you've suddenly got to chase down a wandering child, or you have someone trying to climb you. Lower heels make it easier to stay balanced, and they keep your feet from taking too much abuse.

Then again, sometimes your little one can pull a "Gotcha!" on you when he or she is not even in your presence. I will never forget the night of the infamous "slow speed chase" starring O.J. Simpson, A.C. Cowlings, a white Ford Bronco, and a large cast of police and Highway Patrol cars.

The demands of its coverage stalled us all at the AP bureau for the duration. As was true whenever we were captives of our news story (like on election nights, the L.A. riots, or such disasters as brush fires and earthquakes), the bureau chief arranged for dinner to be brought in. In bulletin-type stories like this one, where none of us dared leave the bureau for even a quick bite to eat, it helped to be able to dash down the hall just a few yards to dig into the Chinese food or pizza or whatever had been provided. This story certainly qualified for catering.

So there I was, sequestered in my on-air booth, wolfing down some barbecued chicken, watching the TV coverage intensely, and waiting for enough of a time window to open up between live shots so I could feed my tape to Washington via satellite. Frozen like an ice sculpture — transfixed by what none of us — even the most hard-bitten, seen-it-all veterans in the newsroom, could believe we were actually witnessing. It was beyond cliff-hanger time. And all of a sudden, BRRRRRRRIIIIIINNNNNNNGGGGGGG!

The outside phone line rang, and I was jolted so hard that my food flew right out of my face. My sauce-covered chicken leg fairly jumped from my grasp, and of course, right down the middle of my nice beaded blouse. On the other end of the line was Mikey, up late on a Friday night, with breaking news of his own: "Momma! I made poo-poo in the toilet!"

Just one more reason why one of my children's many honorary pairs of godparents may be my dry cleaners.

Tips 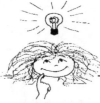 To Remember

✓ Your good work clothes and your child do not make good companions. So you'll have to take precautions.

✓ You may have to temporarily retire some of your better things until your child is a little older and tidier.

✓ In the meantime, you can stay fashionable with accessories — especially one-of-a kind finds.

✓ When you first come home from work, change out of your work clothes AS QUICKLY AS POSSIBLE. Power suits, high heels, and light-colored fabrics are not kid friendly, and your kid will be eager to get friendly with you now that you're home. Also, take off your makeup if you can.

✓ Put on SOMETHING THAT CAN TAKE PUNISHMENT. Preferably kept within easy reach — in case you come under siege. Scan your child's face for dirt or goop, and his or her hands for same. Also check what he or she might be holding that could do damage.

✓ Be aware of where you'll be sitting down — because it may be wearing a kid-mess that will get on you. The mess may or may not be edible.

✓ Prepare to become well-acquainted with the laundry room. Try to stay on top of what is going into which load.

✓ Scan your newly-laundered clothes for stray socks. Especially the itty-bitty ones.

✓ Be on clothes-watch when you're at the office and get a phone call from home. Make sure you're not too dangerously close to something that will mess you up — if the call from home contains a surprise!

Chapter 7
The Mother Of All Battles

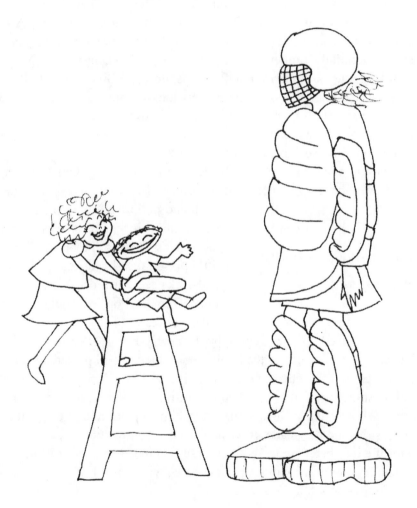

You've heard the old expression about "girding your loins?" As a working mom, you may not be familiar with it, or come to identify with it. You will LIVE AND BREATHE it. Self-defense concerns will demand that you do so. You may come to feel almost like a Secretary of Defense, as a matter of fact!

As much as you may enjoy power-suiting it, with a kid around, you will be most comfortable and battle-ready in around-the-house-and-neighborhood wear. And shoes. Definitely. Something easy to slip on — AND protective.

Like going barefoot around the house, do you? Give it up. Or, if you're into no shoes in the house to keep the carpets looking nice, at least wear slippers. And preferably NOT anything flimsy. It's for your own good, believe me. Having a little person in your life means you now live in a house that's booby-trapped. He or she is a world-class designer of obstacle courses.

Our home has been overrun by liquid-filled teething rings (boy, can they be an adventure when stepped upon and popped), rattles (whole and partially disassembled), push-and-pull toys, little Matchbox cars, Barbie shoes, paintbrushes, broken Crayons, remnants of last week's Cheetos and this morning's Cheerios, little plastic fuse-beads and jacks from the ball-and-jacks set, hard, dried-up clots of Play-doh, Pog slammers, Popsicle sticks and pipe cleaners.

Having a little person in your life means you now live in a house that's booby-trapped.

And they are found in all the darnedest places!

I was tripped up one evening by the nearly-invisible string from a balloon that had been stretched across the family room floor. After I picked myself up, I decided I'd better find the other end of the string so I could dispose of the whole works before someone tried to chew up part of the balloon or use it for bubble gum, and maybe choke on it. I followed the string along the rug, and up the wall to the window sill just behind the shade. It was attached to the balloon's remains, all right, plus part of a half-eaten apple, both carefully wrapped in a pair of little socks, stuffed into the corner of the window, and covered with a nice little swarm of ants. And for who knows how long?

These things are guaranteed to UN-pleasantly surprise you, and your feet, whether you're on active lookout for them or not. They're as inevitable as dirty diapers (which sometimes have mysterious ways of straying from the diaper pail or wastebasket and winding up on the floor). One friend of mine, who neglected to look before leaping, stepped the wrong way, full weight and barefoot — on the very peak of a Barbie boob one night, and the result was a broken ankle. Books — remarkable how sharp and pointy the corners of a book cover can be, no matter how thin the book is. Watch out for candy wrappers; they are as likely to have some of the candy still in them as they are to be empty. And there's the flat stuff too. The smears and stains and stickies. Little spots or blobs on the linoleum in the bathroom or kitchen that are unidentified and almost always gummier than beach tar.

We dare not forget the bigger obstacles — furniture that mysteriously moves — either WAY out of place, or just barely enough to surprise, and break the first stray toes passing by — usually YOURS. Things like step-stools and ottomans and such that your tike will decide are great for pushing around. As I write this, both my husband and I have been left limping for days because Mikey's already in the redecorating business. Do you really want to put your poor feet through all that?

And often, it will be in the dark and the last thing you'll be doing is scanning the floor just ahead of you for obstacles. We've found it necessary to install night-lights as standard equipment in EVERY room of the house. The best ones are those that can operate in emergency mode on batteries when the power goes off. But even this smart step can't always safeguard every one of yours.

Trust me. Save yourself the grief and the Band-Aids or worse. Just make sure you wear shoes. If possible, with rubber soles, which helps immensely when you're dashing across an uncarpeted floor that has surprise wet spots on it, or plastic grocery bags like my son occasionally littered the house with, or the slick paper strips that used to have stickers on them. That way you're less likely to slip and fall and crack your head open. Or slam your hand against the kitchen sink as I did one Sunday morning, trying to break my fall, after racing in, unaware that Mikey had just slimed the floor with pickle relish. That sent me straight to the emergency room and several days of disability leave.

I recall another truly delightful episode, struggling to stretch a pair of my don't-you-dare-wash-these-in-hot-water trousers back out to normal length, because I hadn't found out 'til too late that I'd thrown them in with a load of kids' underwear. After I'd pulled and tugged one time too many, I felt this weird popping feeling near my left elbow. And then, a few moments later, PAIN!!! Another trip to the emergency room revealed a torn ligament, which left me with my arm in a sling, and out on another week or so of disability leave. The timing, as always, couldn't have been more perfect. It knocked me out of commission just days before A: the baptism ceremony for both kids in January, '94, B: the L.A. earthquake that happened early the following morning (another big news story), AND C: the *Golden Globe Awards* a few evenings later (a really big news story for my entertainment beat).

My arm was barely venturing back out into active duty by then — at a time when both my kids were suffering withdrawal from not being "uppied" by me (I couldn't lift either of them with one arm), my husband was tired of having to do ALL the diaper changing, and the right side of my body became over-fatigued from having to shoulder all my equipment-toting burdens alone.

And, by the way, surviving that pre-dawn earthquake was a study in near-disasters just at our house and not as a direct result of any earthquake, either. It wasn't the restlessness of Mother Nature that left our family room floor littered with foot and leg-threatening debris. My kids had handled that just fine the night before, thank you very much!

The quake knocked out all the phones and electricity, which left most of the Southland, our neighborhood included, in total darkness (this is when we learned about the benefits of those power-failure night-lights I mentioned a little bit ago). No phones meant I couldn't call the news desk in Washington OR the bureau downtown to give updates or take deployment assignments of any kind. My battery-powered cell phone wouldn't work, either, even though fully charged, so I couldn't sneak a call through that way.

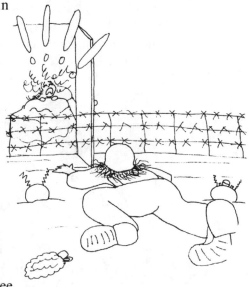

The fearsome shaking woke Elizabeth, who panicked and started screaming for me. I couldn't get to her quickly because Bruce was holding me securely in bed so I'd be safe until the shaking stopped. When it finally did, I had to grope across the house in the direction of her cries. Yes, we had other earthquake supplies, and I had a flashlight with me, but I was in such a hurry to reach Elizabeth that I'd dashed off without my glasses (or, OOPS! shoes). So, even armed with light, I still couldn't see what might lay on the floor ahead of me. Could it be broken glass, or just another Matchbox car?

Once I reached the kids' room, Elizabeth and I huddled together on her bed with the flashlight, listening to a portable radio, while Bruce went outside with another flashlight with our next door neighbors to inspect for leaking gas. Mikey, meanwhile, slept through the entire adventure.

There's one other realization I've come to with no small amount of amusement. It dawned on me awhile ago that every possible substance that can be excreted from any part or orifice of the human body can AND WILL wind up on you after children have come into your life. From ear-wax to tears to runny nose juice and then some! I have been peed on, pooped on, projectile-vomited on, bled on, and let's not forget the ever-popular pus, too. And in all of these cases, the very LAST thing you'll want to do is take care of whatever just got on you. First, you deal with whatever it is that the little person just did and needs as a result. THEN, sometime later, after all the hysteria has died down, you get around to you. See why being messed up has to be okay?

Just bring on the Bactine and Band-Aids, the ointments of every color and consistency, and all available pain relievers with and without aspirin for all the life forms among you. And don't forget the laundry soap and stain remover for everything else. Spot removers, too, for the carpet and furniture and sheets and tablecloths and other things that also have to weather kid-storms. You may want several kinds. And you want to HAVE THEM, period! It's a huge pain realizing too late that what you need most is a fast trip to the 24-hour market for what you forgot you'd run out of. You'll want to keep a spot remover manual in a handy place, right along with your list of poison antidotes and other critical household info.

DO NOT under any circumstances get casual about these things, or forget to keep them almost literally under lock and key. All those horror stories you've heard are based on fact, and illustrate clearly why child-proof caps, and some of those drawer and cabinet safety gizmos may be annoying, but are vital.

I've hit upon another stunning realization — or rather, it hit me. And continues to do so to this day. Never mind the punishment my kids give my clothes — there are times when I'd arrive at work in the morning with brand new mementos from them on my body. This is another one of those issues that no one ever thinks to warn you about in advance. It can happen a lot. And even though I'm well aware of it now, it still comes as a surprise every time.

Your sweet little angel can give you a devil of a rough time. Early-on with each of my two, I developed this nearly constant ache in my head. Not a headache per se. The persistent pain of having your hair pulled constantly. Many a new mom has learned to switch to short hair, updo or pony-tail for a new hairstyle, to get her hair away from baby's hands. Babies are a lot like koalas and opossums, clinging to their mother's fur to stay onboard.

Not only that, but both my babies could wield their heads like mallets from the very beginning, even while they didn't yet have an ounce of control over their movements or any realization of what or who or where they were. Even to this very moment, they still don't know their own strength. And since you'll tend to hold them a lot and hover within easy kissing range, it's inevitable that you'll get thwunked.

I've forgotten by now how many times I've been bashed in the face, the nose, the lip, the eye, and all parts of the head. You suppose it's brain damage or something? They've each rocketed up from below at different times and bonked me under the chin, and I've darn near chomped off the sides of my tongue as a result. I've had my ears yanked and screamed into, fingers poked in my eyes, my skin raked by sharp little fingernails, my legs stood upon, my feet and my hands stomped on, my neck nearly dislocated as one or both of them tries to climb aboard, or swing from, every time I bend over, and every part of my body has been thoroughly kneed and elbowed. I'm convinced by now that small children shouldn't even be issued elbows until they're in grade school. Mikey, in particular, has been a "mis-guided muscle" since he first drew breath.

I know some women whose noses have visibly changed shape since they became moms. Far too many times the head of that baby came up and hit the bull's-eye, full force, before Mom could duck. Now, that same Mom is seriously considering, and saving up for, plastic surgery. I almost had a tooth knocked out while sitting with Mikey, watching Elizabeth in karate class. He got so excited by what he saw that he careened, head first and full speed, right into my mouth, and connected so powerfully that I could have sworn his last name was Tyson.

The way you patch yourself back together for the outside world is to investigate a good blemish cover-up at the cosmetics counter, maybe line up a reliable dentist close by, and learn to enjoy the snickers you'll get from coworkers when you explain what actually happened. And if you wind up going my friend's route and needing professional help for your nose, just coordinate as best you can with your vacation schedule at work. And reassign a little of your wardrobe savings accordingly.

I regret to tell you I'm a battle-scarred veteran of this by now, and still know of no really effective way to avoid being at least a little banged up. Unless, of course, you decide you'd just rather never get close enough to be touched. And you certainly never EVER retaliate in kind. Just work on your reaction time, keep an ice pack and aspirin handy, and be glad that they're THAT anxious to be near you. Motherhood can be a very vigorous contact sport.

Tips To Remember

✓ The kid who's so rough on clothes will also be rough on you. You'll need your wits about you while close by — or home with — your child.

✓ Casual clothing will render you most battle-ready. As will shoes. Or slippers if you aim to keep your rugs clean.

✓ No matter how you try to keep order, your child can still booby-trap your home in short order, leaving toys around to step on. Both big and small, flat, round, and pointy. Sometimes they move furniture in the way.

✓ Your best bet at being taken by surprise is after dark. Therefore, a flashlight or night light is essential.

✓ Your child has several ways of messing you up. By peeing or pooping on you, crying, bleeding, or vomiting. Keep medical and cleaning supplies current and handy — but NOT so handy as to pose a danger to your kid. Make sure you have spot remover manuals AND poison antidote information handy.

✓ Your priority is ALWAYS to take care of the child's troubles first, before your own.

✓ Your child will play rough with you right from the beginning — blissfully unaware of his or her own strength. You face hair pullings, bonks on the nose, elbows in the ribs, scratches, bites, and pinches, feet stompings, and your ears being screamed into. Mainly because you'll always hover within cuddling range.

✓ Severe mishaps may even require corrective nasal or dental surgery.

Chapter 8

You Want That "To Go"?

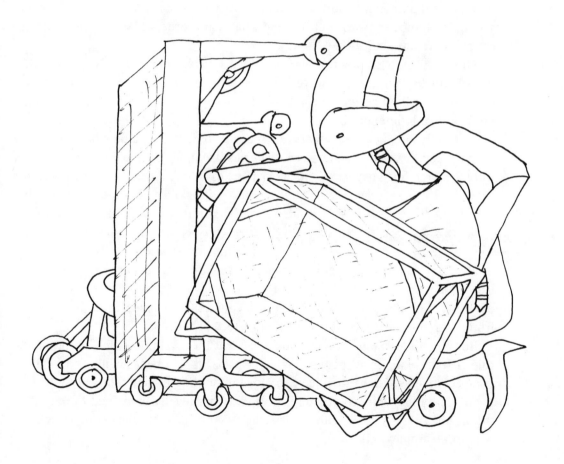

Roll out the heavy artillery, because it's time for troop deployment! It begins, frankly, before you do. You start hearing about the unconditional and mandated-by-law need for a car-seat while you're still pregnant. They won't send your baby home with you from the hospital without one. And they'll fit into any size car, as even Steven Spielberg found out when his first child arrived, and a baby seat became a permanent fixture in his sports car. But there's a whole battery of larger equipment you'll find lumbering into your life, and what spare corners of your house and your car trunk are left undisturbed 'til now.

The arrival of Elizabeth meant not one but two car-seats. No, make that three! My husband and I were both infants, ourselves, on the parenthood growth chart, and so we figured — little baby? Little car-seat, right? Well, yeah, but only temporarily.

The really small car-seats that are a made-to-order fit for a new baby will only fit that nicely for a little while. Because babies inevitably do one thing you're never fully prepared for. They grow. One advantage to an infant-scale car-seat is that it's usually designed with some big across-the-top handle that you can swing overhead. Then you can tote it around with you, outside the car. It also installs and removes easily. So if you have one, enjoy it while it lasts. Another advantage is that you'll use it for a brief enough time that it'll still be in fine condition when it's been outgrown. You can give it away with a clear conscience or expect more great service from it for your next arrival if you think there'll be one.

Babies inevitably do one thing you're never fully prepared for. They grow.

But your little one will be needing a car-seat for a long time. In California, the rule is four years or 40 pounds. Which means, if you began with one of those compact models, you'll soon have to move up to the full-size sedan version. Any good, sturdy one will last you until your child has legally graduated from it. And the big ones usually come with padded adapters to bulk up the insides so a tiny child won't flop around in it.

But a few moments ago, I did say we had three car-seats, including that first little beginner's-sized one. When we realized we were about to outgrow it, we graduated to the upgrade. But almost immediately, we discovered that even THIS step wasn't quite sufficient.

You can expect to use more than one car-seat because it'll soon become clear to you that you really need one PER car. You'll start out thinking you can just switch it from your car to his car and back, as needed. But I guarantee you, just one or two times struggling with that will be enough to convince you that you don't need the grief, the grunting, the groaning, or the muscle strain. The darn thing goes on the back seat and it's usually just big enough NOT to slide right into place easily. Olympic Greco-Roman wrestling is easier than this!

You'll also come to appreciate a stroller. Maybe even a fleet of them! Around our house, there soon appeared several collapsible models called umbrella strollers — smaller, simpler, fewer moving parts, and oh, yes, don't forget, one per car. And a third one in the front hall closet for brief jaunts if you don't want to have to be running to the garage and fumbling with car trunk keys for your original one, while at the same moment, your "Tasmanian Devil" is careening around you at full throttle. Then we got one of those standard-size jobs for the daily walk around the neighborhood. After awhile it got so beaten up by "Introductory Kid" wanting to stand on it, climb all over it, and ride on its roof, that it had to be replaced.

By then, "Second Kid" arrived and we decided to try a two-fer. Those come in several models and sizes, where they ride side-by-side or one behind the other. The first is annoyingly wide and cumbersome but avoids arguments, because both get the front seat. The second is less annoyingly wide, but can cause some bickering because there's room in the front seat for only one. This stroller is quite long and many versions of it have an adjustable back seat that allows the rear passenger to

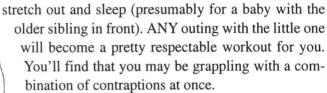

stretch out and sleep (presumably for a baby with the older sibling in front). ANY outing with the little one will become a pretty respectable workout for you. You'll find that you may be grappling with a combination of contraptions at once.

Here's something else I gained new respect for after colonizing Planet Baby: purse size. I'm used to larger purses because my radio reporting job often required having a tape recorder, mike and cables, spare cassettes, batteries, and pens, note pads, my datebook and other tools with me. When little people came into my life that big purse graduated from convenience to necessity. Prepare to add at least some of what I'm about to list to your bag-of-all-trades. Unless you'd prefer to add another bag, entirely, which for short trips will be more of a hassle than you already have. And just to make it clear, I'm talking about brief runs away from home. You'll have to compound all this accordingly, if you're considering something more substantial — from an overnight away to a week's vacation.

Then again, maybe you'd rather just throw up your hands and go rent a U-Haul.

Bag-of-all-Trades

Diapers (either cloth or disposable). Or pull-ups, depending on the age of the leakiest little one. One or two depending on the length of your trip.

Babywipes in a small Zip-Lock Bag. During as well as after the diaper era, they still clean like gangbusters. I keep a separate container of them in my car as standard equipment, along with a large box of Kleenex. And yes, I did learn to bag Babywipes. You'll sometimes see small plastic cases in the store, designed for portability and convenience. But I have found that these don't have a tight seal. Whatever wipes are in there will soon dry out and thus be unusable. Those little individually-wrapped wipes are nice, but you may find them to be somewhat impractical. You'll probably need one RIGHT NOW! And you won't have the time or patience to fiddle with any hermetically-sealed little foil wrappers.

Three or four crayons and paper. They keep a kid occupied while in the waiting room, the restaurant, the church pew, the car, the bus, whatever. Little spiral notepads are fine. Both my kids loved my official Reporters Notebooks, and I'd wind up having to guard them with my life. Or else, I'd be at some news conference, furiously taking notes, and suddenly find myself out of clean paper because the rest of the pages in the pad had all these waxy, multi-colored doodles all over them.

One or two small Zip-Lock Bags containing a snack. Dry kid-type cereals, cookies, crackers, or celery and carrot strips, or string cheese in little single serving packages are best, and the least messy, plus something to drink because they'll be thirsty, too. I recommend apple juice. Repeat, apple juice. Why? Any other kind of juice, when spilled (and inevitably it will be) will stain the car, the kid, and/or you. Apple juice spills you can't see as easily. Milk is too sticky and perishable if left out for any length of time. And NO GUM! You don't need the grief unless they're older and can be counted on NOT to swallow it, stick it onto, or rub it into anything. Or apply it to their hair.

A small toy. Optional, and preferably one without a lot of extra parts. Or a book. But nothing the little one can't live without in case it gets lost. Maybe you'll want to keep this strictly in the car.

One or two empty Zip-Lock Bags, or plastic grocery bags. Kids love picking up treasures from nature walks and other outdoor activities. Virtually anything, even if it's stinky, slimy, or sticky, you're thus able to take home.

I mentioned a bit about keeping supplies in the car. I first was tipped off about this from Joanna Kerns, who learned it, herself, as a mom and as the star of a TV movie about earthquakes. Living in earthquake country, as I described earlier, means our house already had a fairly respectable stockpile of emergency supplies. But she wised me up about extending that preparedness to the car, as well.

I stow a sports bag in the trunk with some worst-case-scenario essentials in it. Expanded ever so slightly, you'll be well-equipped for "Typhoon Tike."

I've always kept a blanket in the car for warmth. Actually, it's no blanket at all, but rather an ankle-length woolen poncho that I have been known to throw on when I'd get stuck out late on assignment. Like the services for Martha Raye, which were SUPPOSED to take an hour or two in the late afternoon, but really continued on well after dark. Or the memorial to Dinah Shore, during which we reporters were kept outside, in the cold, AND soon enough also, not only in the dark, but in the rain. It's big enough to handle my creature discomforts, and better yet, it also covers two sets of little legs in the back seat when two little sets of mouths start whimpering about being cold. And it doesn't look too disgusting just thrown onto the back seat.

We working mothers are also charter members of the Corner-Cutters' Club.

An old beach towel or bath towel is a must. Even if it winds up being stomped into a mound on the floor of the back seat. Just wait until you have to sop up some spill before it seeps down into your seat springs!

A water bottle. One of those clear ones you can find in any grocery store. They come in multiple liter sizes. Most importantly, they have those little caps whose tops lift up with the brisk motion of one hand (your other hand will be on the steering wheel in heavy traffic!) or even between your teeth. Yeah, I know, we've all been urged not to use our teeth for such things, but we working mothers are also charter members of the Corner-Cutters' Club. Water will squirt out fairly harmlessly through a small hole in the middle of the top. When finished, you just push the little movable top back down and it clicks shut. A kid who's grown into semi-responsible age, as the remarkable Elizabeth was at three-and-a-half or so, can learn to operate it for you.

My earthquake kit in the trunk also contains a small first-aid kit. A simple one that you can find at the drug store and stash away for time of need. I've also got a mini-version in a small Zip-Lock Bag that will fit in my purse or glove compartment. It contains about four to six Band-Aids, a traveler's size bottle of children's Tylenol or other pain reliever — either via dropper or chewable tablet as they get older, and maybe a small tube of ointment. My husband's always been really big on Neosporin. I also keep small bottles of Bactine and children's sunblock in the trunk.

The earthquake kit in the trunk also has nonperishable num-nums for sustenance in a pinch. Things like bags of nuts, raisins, trail mix, and hard candy — quick-fix energy boosters with a long shelf-life, so they won't go stale if left in there for months. Invariably, some little person will wind up hungry on even a brief road trip, in an area where snack stops aren't possible or available.

For those who REALLY want to be prepared, one of those little "quick-n-dirty" inexpensive cameras is nice to stash in the trunk. Truly, you can't predict when you'll be driving somewhere with offspring when an inspiration hits you — to go to the park, or someplace that catches your eye as you pass. Maybe if it's wintry where you are, you have to stop for a few minutes and make a snowman. Or you'll have to go stomp on some sand at the beach or seashore if you're in that area. You'll inevitably find yourself regretting that you don't have a camera handy when he or she does something REALLY cute. Or silly. Photogenic in any case. Keep one in your "bag of all trades" and you'll never have to worry about that.

Deidre Hall told me after one interview that she went so far as to install those little cheap-o cameras in EVERY room of her house, let alone in the car. That way, she knew she wouldn't miss any of those little one-time-only photo-ops that she'd want to record for posterity. It works beautifully, although you do have to be savvy about where you stash the camera. Fingers far smaller than yours are sure to find it and have their way with it, too, unless you take care. But this scheme does prevent your having to race off to find the camera, and then fumble with it, and hope there's still film in it, only to find that your munchkin's adorable little Kodak moment is long gone.

I've also found it handy to keep one or two trash bags in the trunk. They can function simply as trash bags (or other), since your little person will generate unfathomable amounts of litter for you. How about waterproofing for the back seat of the car? I discovered this when my daughter surprised me after kindergarten one day with the class rabbit. She'd earned the privilege of taking it home for the night. Count on said rabbit to pee on the way home, which it did, in our case. It went on the trashbag covering the seat, and NOT the seat itself.

PORT-A-
mom

That's also why I was grateful that I hadn't removed a couple of day's worth of newspapers from the floor of the back seat of the car. (See, sometimes it's good to be a slob!) I'd layered them on top of the trashbag, and they absorbed the rabbit juice. (Always did appreciate those editorials!)

The trashbags have additional uses in being able to prevent little fannies from getting wet, or dampening the car, or you. If they've been to the beach. If they just spilled something, or had an — um — accident. If they want to go sit on the grass and IT'S wet, and you'd like them to stay dry. OR, if you all get caught in a rain shower and have to make a run for it. They can be draped over the tops of your heads like a tarp, or with a hole cut in the middle of the bottom, and both bottom corners, you then have head and hand holes — and an instant rain slicker.

And mind you, YOU have it. You need to supervise this one CLOSELY. **Plastic Bags Aren't Toys!** But they can be very useful tools when handled judiciously. Just make sure you're vigilant about this, and consider it strictly as a last resort.

Did I just say newspapers? My AP job always left me with a few on the floor of the back seat or trunk of my car. Those newspapers are great for emergencies. Like the rabbit episode. Or, when you are out running errands on a hot day and unable to find your windshield sun-screen. I've been known to drape a section of newspaper over the top of my steering wheel, so it won't fry my hands.

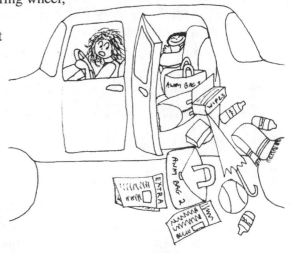

Another section covered Mikey's baby seat in the back, because even if you haven't lost that windshield sunscreen, and/or you don't mind fumbling with it, it IS for the FRONT only. No matter how you park, or how carefully you search for a shady spot, the sun moves and you'll return to find the car-seat right out there — fully unprotected and ready to cook a nice egg upon. I briefly tried fastening the seat closed so it would be at its smallest mass with the least amount exposed to the heat of the sun. But then, when we were ready to get back in the car, loaded with packages, who needed all that extra fumbling to get the car-seat open again? So I'd leave it open and cover it, and it would stay cooler.

By the way, a moment like this also calls for that bottle of water you stashed in the car, too. All right, so it's drinking water. It's also cool. And in a fix, it can be squirted onto the hot baby seat before it touches that little skin. The babywipes also come in handy here, too, because their moisture is equally cooling.

Other additionals for the car, if you have the time and/or budget to throw them in:

Cassettes. Of all kinds. Their favorite popular music, classical music to educate and edify, or story readings. Try recording your own because your voice is soothing and familiar. For longer trips, songs with vocals let you all get creative and make up your own verses. We've invented some that are fairly gross and disgusting, wildly and wickedly amusing to the little people who dreamed them up, and are guaranteed to yield some very cheery young travelers. For older kids, comedy tapes, provided they're not crammed full of swear words. For the more financially high-fallutin' out there, the car CD player and corresponding accouterments apply here.

There's one other VERY valuable extra in this department. You'll soon discover that car rides can lull even the feistiest little person right down into a nice nap. So this is when you can cheat a bit, and get some extra work done. Now's the time to pop in that cassette of the business seminar during which you wish you'd taken notes. You might decide to tape one of your staff meetings and play it back here. If a helpful colleague has taped one you missed or had interrupted, you've got a chance to catch up.

You'll soon discover that car rides can lull even the feistiest little person right down into a nice nap.

I kept pace on quite a few interview sessions using that system, and once actually completed a cut-sheet on a 25-minute Kevin Bacon Q-and-A, including quote details, with a kid dozing in the baby seat behind me. Or try one of those learn-a-foreign-language tapes. It might work subliminally on your snoozing little one while you're boning up, too.

Some working moms I know choose this time to use their pocket recorders to dictate notes to themselves. Nobody else is awake and hollering or jabbering right then, or trying to grab it from you because it looks like a neat new toy.

Kids clothes. I learned to keep a spare change or two in the trunk. Something they can put on if they aren't dressed warmly enough, or get wet, like a sweater or sweatshirt. Also take something lighter in case if they're too hot. A change of shoes, extra socks and underwear. All these can be simplified and adjusted according to seasonal needs. And if I even slightly suspect we'll be out later than usual, I'll throw in a pair of pajamas for each of them. I've found it's smarter to change them into their pajamas while you're away — BEFORE they doze off. That way, they're totally bed-ready and won't wake up after you get home while you're fumbling with their PJ's. Then, astonishingly enough, you actually have the rest of the evening to yourself!

With a little person in your life, sooner or later you'll find out the hard way that you'll need most if not all of the supplies I've mentioned. Having them handy will equip you to handle almost all unscheduled rabbits and other misadventures. What I've had to keep in the car usually winds up cluttering only the floor of the back seat, right in front of the baby seat when we had one. It IS confinable. Nevertheless, I found that the buildup on the floor in front of the baby seat also raised the floor level a bit, providing my son with an instant step-stool when he needed it.

If you have one or more little ones, it will be an ongoing challenge to maintain order.

Okay, I admit it, my car is not in pristine condition most of the time. But if you have one or more little ones, it will be an ongoing challenge to maintain order, whether you have any problem-solving supplies with you or not. Besides, I stow the REALLY heavy artillery in the trunk. I'll trade a little clutter for instant disaster repellent any day. And as they get older, I'll get even. Cleaning and/or washing my car on a regular basis just might wind up being one of the chores THEY can do.

There IS one more very critical element to completing this package if you REALLY want it to be as fail-safe as possible.

If you can afford it, a **cellular phone** is invaluable. Not only is it convenient, but it can be a life-saver. Particularly if you suddenly have to call the Auto Club and you can't — or you'd rather not have to look for a pay phone. As you settle in on Planet Baby, you may find this is yet another objective toward which you'll decide to re-direct some of your extra wardrobe money.

I also found that the **beeper** my job demanded I wear at all times also served my husband. He beeped me much more often than the assignment desk ever did. Still does, too, because we got our own beeper system after I said farewell to the needs of that particular assignment desk. Sometimes it's just to say "hi." At other times it's to relay an important message about juggling client appointments and school pickup times, or having to race someone to the emergency room RIGHT NOW! If you don't have to have a beeper for work, you may find it worthwhile to get one for home — for kid-management. Another for your spousal unit, for two-way communication. Your offspring will eventually want and need your beeper number, also.

Beepers can be great! Worth their weight in platinum! And even in cases when you think they're exactly the opposite. Having that beeper interface between home and work has been a fabulous "cover-your-you-know-what" device on several occasions for me. Considering that my AP job kept me on a LOOOOOOOOONNNNNNNGGGGGGG leash from my supervisor in Washington, I'd check in, in the morning, and THEN proceed into the rest of my day. And occasionally, I'd take advantage of a slow morning to take my young 'uns to the doctor or out to a burger brunch or something — then go into the bureau for the routine stuff later in the day.

Of course, this most perfect of back-stopping systems did break down on rare occasion (and by the way, you can expect this to happen, as each and every most-perfect of back-stopping systems has a divinely-decreed right to do).

Naturally, one of those was the day when Roseanne and her then-husband Tom Arnold called a surprise news conference about some paparazzi run-in, with one hour's notice. Early-on, no one had a clue about what Roseanne's camp might have up its sleeves for later in the day. First thing in the morning it looked like the coast was clear. So my husband and I decided that — since it was a REALLY slow newsday, and I'd already checked in with my supe and HE had nothing for me, and I had no assignments pre-scheduled — we'd just put off getting too dressed up, and use part of the morning to take the little people on a drive. Makes perfect sense, doesn't it? And, after all, I'd thoroughly checked and double-checked all possible schedules and assignment desk rundowns first.

We got just a few miles up the freeway when my beeper went off, and by the time I could get to a phone, the irate voices from Washington informed me that Roseanne and Tom were right that minute in the middle of things and Washington had been trying to beep me to dispatch me there for an hour.

After I scraped my stomach off the floor of the car, we raced for home so I could throw on some respectable work clothes and grab my gear, and off I went to cover Roseanne and Tom. I arrived just in time to play some serious, major league catch-up, but the assignment got covered.

And you know what? It turned out QUITE OK, believe it or not. How come? Because that beeper automatically left a trail of electronic bread crumbs that could be used to find me a way out of that mess. The no-longer-irate UPPER-LEVEL voices from Washington were able to determine that there had been a power failure at our local beeper service company, precisely at the time they'd been trying to send me to Roseanne and Tom. Therefore, my beeper had been knocked out of commission. In addition, since I didn't have a cell phone assigned to me at the time, more precious minutes were lost while I searched for an off ramp with a working pay phone attached reasonably closeby, I wound up with further ammunition to argue successfully to be better-equipped.

However, even Roseanne herself wasn't influential enough to finally get me a cell phone for sure. It still took an after-hours earthquake in the middle of my drive home at the end of a long day (which meant I had to find a safe place to pull off to find a phone, so I could be sent back to the office to work the story on overtime), AND one of the visiting managers from Washington with a rental car before they agreed to authorize a cell phone for me. Still, combined mishaps like these did ultimately build me a convincing case for one, and it's served me, my work, AND my Mommy track, ever since.

Many's the time that combined beeper-and-cell phone system kept people happy on both ends of my priority spectrum. I was in the middle of an interview with Dennis Farina one day in the middle of January, 1991, when my beeper went off. Ordinarily I'd hold off responding 'til the interview or whatever I was in the midst of was over. But glancing down at it, I could see the number read-out was the emergency code that Bruce and I had figured up for our own private use. I begged Farina's pardon, excused myself, and called home. "Mary! Did you hear? They're bombing Baghdad!" The assignment desk hadn't called me since this kind of thing wasn't exactly my beat. But it seemed like a VERY good idea to check in anyway, since all of us, especially on the understaffed broadcast end, had been looking at contingency plans in case things grew really nasty in the Persian Gulf.

As it turned out, this WAS a most auspicious time to check in, and the folks back at the home office were happy to hear from me. They told me to go right home, but stay close by my beeper, in case things had to be shuffled but good in the next few hours. And Dennis Farina proved himself to be a most understanding gent about it, especially since he'd been following the news closely, himself, and wasn't surprised that I'd have to cut our interview short.

The drive home, as I recall, was filled with beeper traffic. Bruce beeped again. Washington did, again. Even my coworker at the L.A. bureau (who was just about to be dispatched east, to the Pentagon) got in touch, just to make sure I was reachable in the event I would have to cover HIS beat if he left.

And that's exactly what happened, by the way.

Also, it was very helpful to be beepable when the emergency was not in the news, but at home. My beeper went off while I was out on assignment one morning. It was Bruce. "Mary, can you come home in the next few hours? Something's come up." He never resorted to this type of request unless there was no other alternative. "Where are you right now?" My response: "Covering a Pee-wee Herman rally outside CBS." (Pee-wee was in the doghouse with the network at the moment, because his real-life alter-ego had been caught in a Florida adult theater, and fans in L.A. were showing their loyalty.) Bruce was far from our house with a client he couldn't break free from, and our baby-sitter who didn't drive needed to leave to deal with a personal problem at home.

What followed, after wrapping up in the field, was a race back to the bureau to package the story fully and properly, finish everything else that I could, and head home to help address everyone's needs.

You always have to remember the care and feeding of a beeper and cell phone system, though, and make it part of your nightly routine. I make it a habit to park my cell phone in its charger at the end of every day. Once a month, the beeper batteries need to be changed. And you HAVE to stay on top of this. As easily-manageable as it appears, you have no idea how often little details like this get overlooked, and then you're guaranteed to find yourself sunk, but good, at the worst possible time.

I also have to stay on top of everything else that I'd stashed in the car, to keep mishaps of all kinds to a minimum. For example, you have to regroup with the kids' extra clothes that now need washing and recycling, or retiring (you'll be amazed how rapidly they're outgrown). Towels and such that are wet. Snacks and stuff in my purse that have to be extracted just so I won't get grossed out. Like the bananas my son always loves, but only seems to want half of. You know how easily even a nice, fresh, solid banana can be reduced to slush.

And of course, there is the ever-present embarrassment factor to try to avoid. I remember covering a big news conference with Michael Jackson's family, who fielded a bajillion questions about child molestation allegations while he was overseas on a world tour. Serious stuff. I too, had a few questions to ask them. At the end, a few of us from various media outlets compared notes before we headed back to our respective bureaus. I had to reach into my purse to get a business card, but first (and in front of these people, mind you) had to pull out a couple of spare diapers left over from a recent day trip with the kids. Seems I'd forgotten to clear them out after the excursion had ended.

You may have noticed an overriding theme to this entire chapter. Whenever you want to go somewhere with your kid, spontaneity goes, too. As in — goes AWAY.

Tips To Remember

✓ More items of larger size will be moving into your home once a baby has. Particularly those pertaining to kid transport.

✓ The first one you'll need is a carseat (mandatory as of the ride home from the hospital). They vary according to size, age, and purpose, so consider the specific needs of your child now, and in the months/years ahead.

✓ You'll also need a stroller, perhaps a simple one to start — for the cost and portability. You may have to replace it with a more complex variety, depending on the size, age, and number of children.

✓ The size of your purse may change.

✓ Unless you plan to use a separate bag just for child necessities, you may want to upgrade to a larger purse.

✓ Because you'll HAVE to take at least a small amount of supplies along for ANY trip of ANY length with a kid. Particularly a young one. How much you want to have with you depends on the length and nature of the trip. This mainly to car trips.

✓ You'll need to have with you: Spare diapers (for changes), Babywipes (for cleaning up), crayons and paper, or a small toy or book (for amusement), snacks and drinks, an empty plastic bag or Zip-Lock Bag — to contain anything — clean OR messy, that may need to be taken home by your child (or you).

✓ You'll need to adapt the above for the trunk of your car — so you're equipped to handle emergencies.

- ✓ Necessary items include a blanket (for warmth), an old beach or bath towel (for drying or sopping), a water bottle, a plastic trash bag or two (for waterproofing and containment), flashlight, first-aid kit, and non-perishable snacks. Also consider a change of clothes and shoes for your child (for warmth and cleanliness).

- ✓ A small inexpensive camera is also good to have along, just in case.

- ✓ Items from the trunk that work just as well in the passenger area:

- ✓ A blanket (for coverage and warmth), a newspaper for coverage, sopping, or sun/heat shielding.

- ✓ You have to stay on top of your supplies:

- ✓ Non-perishable food and drinks can not be kept for long.

- ✓ Dirty items need cleaning and replacing.

- ✓ Spare clothes and shoes will be outgrown if kept for long. In the very least, they'll probably need laundering.

- ✓ Any diapers or other items in your purse should be removed after the trip is over, so they won't get in your way at work.

- ✓ Your car may be cluttered — only for awhile — and when your child is older, he or she can help you clean it up.

- ✓ Make technology your friend. It'll help you manage kids and stay connected.

- ✓ Many time-saving gadgets are available to assist.

- ✓ Music or comedy cassettes in the car can be used for child amusement. Make your own by recording your own story readings. Same with CD's.

- ✓ Music in the car can also lull your child to sleep so you can: catch up on work, listen to seminar tapes or other work-related recordings. Perhaps some made by a colleague of a meeting you missed.

✓ Make sure your child remains seated in back if you have equipment installed in front (like cell phones or mobile fax machines).

✓ Cellular phones are good tools for staying in contact — with spouse, home, kids, and office.

✓ A beeper system goes hand-in-hand with a cell phone, so you'll know who wants to make contact with you. Your kid will eventually want to join the system, too.

✓ Don't forget to maintain these tools. Cell phones need regular recharging, and beepers need a battery change every month.

✓ Your growing family will force your space needs to grow too — so you may soon need a substantial gadget: a larger car.

Chapter 9

Whine With Dinner

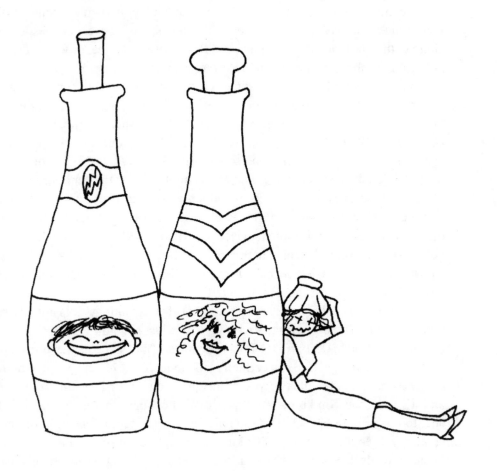

"**C**are for a little wine?" my friend Annie Lockhart cheerfully asked when we were all out at a big neighborhood picnic together. "No, thanks," said I with a sigh, "I already have two."

I have quite literally dined out on that joke for some time now. If you have one or more munchkins in your life, you'll come up with your own version. Up 'til now, your dinners out have probably been with friends, business colleagues, or just you alone with your mate in some quiet, candle-lit corner. A nice, orderly, adult dinner. All of that changes radically when Restaurant Row relocates to Planet Baby.

First of all, WHERE you go changes. Having one or more little ones means you're better off going to eateries where it's not out of the ordinary to see little ones. An elegant bistro or steakhouse just may not be it. Sushi bars, especially AT the sushi bar, don't work too well, either (I'm personally grief-stricken to say). Nor would any place you'd take a client on an expense account. Dinner theater? Forget it!

"Care for a little wine?"

Places I was never interested in suddenly zoomed to the top of the list after Elizabeth arrived. Mainly because they had a kid-bar, or balloons, or pink and orange decor, or lots of Formica surfaces and menus with pictures on them. Or better yet, menus to color! Places where the other booths were filled with lots of little squirming arms and legs. Yeah, I know, it's not sophisticated dining, and the atmosphere is non-existent. But it's QUITE kidproof.

Mind you, all of this applies to your own off-duty outings. It is not advisable to take a child to a business dinner with you. You just shouldn't. If you have to go to one of those, you MUST arrange for a baby-sitter. That is, if you plan on maintaining a professional image. You can certainly talk about 'em. But leave 'em at home. The only exception to this rule is if you're meeting a client for, say, lunch or something, and it's someone you know VERY well. Well enough, that is, to know that he or she, too, is a mom or dad. And ONLY if he or she, too, is planning on including small-fry. It could, indeed, be that kind of set-up. For example, I do know of a few business deals that were born to various parents attending the same kids' party.

Become familiar with the verb "to spill." You will learn to conjugate it in more ways than you ever imagined. I quickly made it a habit to take not one napkin from the napkin dispenser, but a whole wad of them. No matter how big a wad I bring back to the table, every last napkin in it is put to good use. Sometimes my supplies have had to be reinforced by the napkin wad Bruce learned to bring back to our table with him.

Everything that can get spilled, be it yours OR your kid's, will get spilled. Drinks of course, and sauces of every kind. And it doesn't even have to be a liquid. You should have seen the floor around any table where we were seated, for several years straight. It looked like we were sitting on a Jackson Pollock painting. As much food wound up on the floor as in their stomachs. Mostly they just dropped it, or maybe had a utensil-control problem. However, I've known babies who've deliberately thrown their food down onto the floor with all their pint-sized might.

Sometimes it isn't even a food item. On a regular basis I used to have to pull sneak-raids on vacant tables near us, for replacement forks and spoons. At home, when we realized the only clean-up crew was US, we took to using a splat-mat under each of their chairs. A sterling sanity saver!

Sometimes they don't bother waiting to get to your table to start spilling. One time we all went to our favorite salad place, where you serve yourself on a tray, as you proceed down a long counter of green, crunchy, veggie-type stuff. I built my usual pile-on-a-plate, with a second smaller plate's worth for my son. He was securely strapped into a rolling kid-seat that the restaurant had as part of its standard equipment (yet another clue that this is a kid-friendly place). I assumed Mikey was "safed."

WRONG!

He was JUST close enough to the counter to reach out to my tray as we approached the end of the line where the cash register was, and he latched on. In one swift movement, the whole works had been pulled over onto the floor. Not to mention all down my leg.

The minute you all sit down, there's a race across the table top to see who can grab the knife first, and of course, the blade end is always preferable! I consistently wound up with EVERYTHING interesting on the table pulled over to my place to keep it out of their reach. And I do mean everything. From the flower vase in the center, or the little candle (which we'd usually move to another table altogether), to the mustard and ketchup caddie, or the oil and vinegar caddie, or the salt and pepper shakers, the little pats of butter on the butter dish (with or without wrappers), the bread they're sure to goof with or shred, or chow down on, so they have no room left in their stomachs for dinner, and DEFINITELY the container with all the little sugar packets.

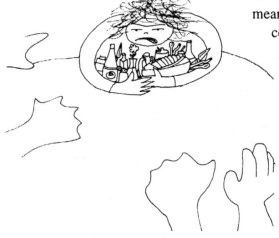

Those really aren't the objects I just described, per se, you know. They're actually toys — to be played with and fought over. That goes double for whatever's inside them. A small wonder that there was ever any room at my place on which to serve food.

Never order the little person a meal of his or her own unless it's kid-sized. The restaurants you'll wind up choosing will usually have a kid menu anyway, and the best ones always supply crayons with it. The little one is guaranteed to want more than he or she will wind up eating.

Sometimes, even now that Elizabeth and Mikey are older, we don't even bother with a kid's serving. We order for ourselves and make sure it's something they'll eat, too. This works quite nicely, provided you're willing to sacrifice a bit on your own menu choices, AND you ask for an extra plate or two. And you're content with not having all of your meal to yourself. Then you can cut off the appropriate amount for your kid, on his or her own private plate. On slow-service nights, you can always use the butter dishes, if such there be. You'll probably 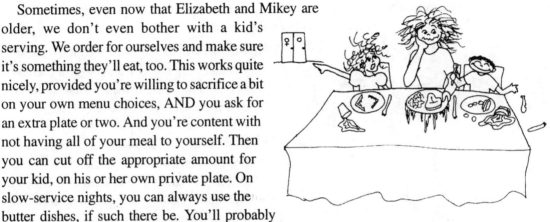 give up part of your dinner in any event, whether you want to or not. Simply because they'll see what you ordered and decide they'd rather have that, instead.

Let me pause here a minute to pose you a question. Do you like cold food? I hope you said yes. If not, you'll have to learn to like it. Because that's how YOUR food will always be by the time YOU get to eat it. Even if it's served still sizzling from the grill.

And what's your opinion about fast food? I'm not talking about some drive-thru burger franchise. I'm talking about the "Beat the Kid's Clock" game you'll play with yourself with every dinner out (and at home, too, for that matter). Motherhood has left me with the nasty habit of wolfing down my meals. Because I'm never sure how long I'll REALLY be permitted to enjoy what I'm eating. Or to really know what it tastes like before some little fingers decide to come dancing and digging and doodling their way in. Or spilling something incompatible into it.

You'll find your meal is short-stopped at the outset, and at the end, and at any arbitrary point in the middle because your favorite little dining companion is constantly in need of something. You won't be allowed to start eating when everybody else at your table does. You never know when you'll have to pause to come to someone's assistance, or for how long, or how many more times after that. And by the time you CAN enjoy a few bites, you're so far behind that everyone else is finished, fidgety, and whining to go home.

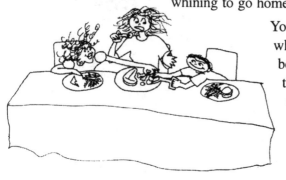

Your tike will come up with umpteen reasons why you can't dig right in, and most of them will be extremely legitimate. You'll have to dish out their portion. Test it to see if it's not too hot. Cut it up into elf-sized pieces (which will help it cool faster). Susan Sarandon commented to us once in an interview session that this was just one of many reasons that made her think twice about having too many more babies. She wondered how old she'd be — before she'd be able to eat a full dinner without having to stop and cut somebody else's meat up for them.

And it goes beyond just custom-tailored meat duty. In the case of mashed potatoes and gravy, or ice cream and chocolate sauce, you'll be expected to stir it into a plasma state of matter that we call "monkey-wunk." TAKE AWAY whatever they're drinking, and isolate it 'til they've eaten something. Ignore the inevitable griping that will ensue. Mine always found it really easy to fill up with milk or water or juice or soda first, before the food arrived. At that point, they were too full to eat anything else. Then, by the time we were leaving the restaurant, they'd start complaining about being starved. Besides, if you do separate them from their beverages, that'll be one thing less that they can spill.

You'll also have several other kinds of hurdles to jump, beyond just the food preparation. There are dropped napkins to retrieve and reinstall. Someone always has to be taken to the bathroom, and until lately, it's always had to be me providing the escort service because Bruce claims the men's room is never as clean as the ladies' room is. Which MAY be true.

And until they're older, they MUST be escorted. They won't be able to reach the sink or faucets for hand-washing purposes (an essential skill you want to make sure they learn) without a boost from a big person. For security's sake, you need to be close at hand while they're taking care of things. You have to make sure only the cold water is turned on, and that they don't make an impulsive (and possibly scalding) grab for the hot water faucet instead.

Not only that, but you HAVE to be on hand to curb their irresistible urges to squat down and peek to see who and what might be of interest in the next stall! Inquiring minds seem to want to know, even at this age! And, of course, once they've done so, that means their hands have just walked all over the floor, and will, without question, need to be washed. Maybe a second time, depending on when they tried to stoop 'n snoop.

For everyone else's sake, they need to be attended by somebody tall enough for other grown-ups to see easily. It will not occur to kids to look before they leap, or skip, or run. And it's seldom EVER walk. Rest assured, it's RUN. And at any moment it might also be backwards. With eyes closed. Which means they're likely to smack right into some hapless waiter with loaded tray held on high, or some unsuspecting diner returning to the table holding an equally-loaded tray.

By the way, the pilgrimage to the bathroom appears to be practically unavoidable, despite all our best efforts to head it off at the pass. The most dedicated advance planning seems to hold no sway. Bruce even took to engaging our home intercom system in this battle, with debatable results. Every time we'd get ready to go out to dinner, we made it part of the routine to send everyone to the bathroom first. So the clarion call would echo through the house — "MAY I HAVE YOUR ATTENTION PLEASE? THIS IS YOUR DADDY SPEAKING. EVERYBODY GO PEE,

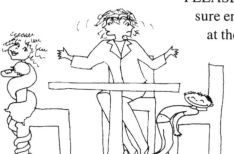

PLEASE! THANK YOU." Well, indeed they would. But sure enough, they'd need to go again after we were seated at the restaurant. About the only solution to this is time. Time for them, AND their bladders, to grow bigger.

All the while you're at table, unless they're firmly strapped into high chairs or special kids' seats, you'll be "kvetching" at them to sit up and sit straight. And hold still! To this day, I'm truly impressed by how many positions a kid can invent while at the table. Well, at least it's usually NEAR the table. If they're shown to a chair, soon they're trying to squeeze underneath it. Or hanging off it by varying degrees. Or kneeling on it. Or squatting. Sideways, or better yet backwards. Sometimes upside down if they're going for broke (or breakage maybe?). And they get extra points if they can do any or all of this while tipping the chair. If you're seated in a booth, the top of the seats is virgin territory worthy of staking a claim upon. And if it's a corner booth, heck, they can even set up a base camp up there.

Or, SAY! Let's go the other way, shall we? Like slumping down 'til they ooze off onto the floor underneath the table. Sometimes taking the chair cushion with them. Naturally, there's a whole new continent down THERE to be explored! And overhead, of course, a new firmament studded with chewing gum splats that need close examination. And don't forget, they've thought ahead to provide food for themselves down there during the adventure. I've occasionally had to threaten to bring along a roll of gaffer's tape with which to tape them into place if they don't straighten up. That usually gets their attention.

However, if there's another kid nearby, especially if it's someone they know, all bets are off. They won't even want to trouble themselves with your table anymore. They'd rather go visiting. Or else have people over. Amazing, isn't it, how much there is to anticipate, here? No management staff strategy meetings I ever attended prepared me for ANY of this.

Sometimes merely sitting still can become your problem. Since Mikey grew old enough to keep it more or less together at restaurants, we've begun venturing into one or two of the better ones on occasion so the kids can field test their table manners. And the very same little boy who was whining and sniveling about being hungry and wanting to go out to dinner just a few minutes before is now stone cold asleep in the middle of the salad plate. Mikey has fallen asleep on the finest table cloths and entrees and most elegant surroundings in our area. And even while his sister is still up and at 'em, creating a commotion. We've conducted all kinds of experiments on the art of propping him up. And we know we're going to wind up carrying him (along with everything else AND his doggie bag) out to the car.

One evening we'd gone to one of those dark, intimate, teensy Italian bistros in the area, and the kids both spotted Bonnie Hunt, whom they'd just seen in *Jumanji*, and I'd interviewed maybe two weeks before. They were thrilled and the restaurant owner offered to take them over to meet her in short order. It wasn't enough to keep Mikey awake, though. By the time we were leaving and passing her table, I was carrying him, and trying desperately to maintain my balance and keep his shoes out of her face as we squeezed through the narrow spaces between tables to say hello.

Be ready for "The Look." I'm certain you'll want to be a dedicated disciple of discipline. But sometimes the kid will just keep pushing that ol' envelope 'til all its corners are punched clean through. You'll be at wit's end. And there will be those seated around you who will make it clear that they are, as well.

I regularly confess, I was one of those who'd have to stifle an urge to glare at some poor souls with kids who were screaming, mewling, hurling, and behaving as if they were in a moon bounce, and not at a proper dinner table in public. "What's wrong with those people?" I'd mumble. "Can't they curb their kids?!" True, some people ARE lax about their parenting. They're the ones who — if you ask "Who's running this joint, you or a three-year-old?"— would blissfully defer to their little people. Don't wanna rain on that three-year-old self-esteem or anything, right? But plenty of others ARE out there valiantly fighting the good fight, and are still coming up losers.

The only answer for this is patience. For me, it was more like being patient for all those years 'til I became a mom. Only then could I know, and be capable of finding a little sympathy in my heart. Those hapless souls are to be saluted and supported. Bruce has even gone so far as to throw them an encouraging comment or two, about how well they seem to be coping, and how we sure took our turns in that barrel, oh-so-recently.

"Who's running this joint, you or a three-year-old?"

You have to try to keep the upper hand, though. Bruce and I both believe that the only things that should be coddled to any great degree are eggs. We've found ourselves trying a version of what I once heard Dr. Laura Schlessinger recommend on the radio: throwing 20 or 30 dollars on the table, picking everybody up bodily, and LEAVING, even sometimes before our order comes. If he or she is old enough to reason with, your little one will get the message if you reinforce that a few times. Obey, or no stay.

If your little one is so little that you can't yet reason with him or her, and it gets REALLY bad (really: LOUD!), you may just have to excuse both of yourselves and go outside for awhile to allow everybody else's ears in the restaurant to stop ringing. They might also have broken glass to clean up following that last high note your screaming infant hit — when you all heard for yourselves that it WAS live, it wasn't Memorex!

We had one trip to a neighborhood eatery that was interrupted by one of the young guests of one of our kids. This little person decided the windows by our table needed washing, and proceeded to stand on the chair and lick them. And after that, the drapes on said windows needed to be adjusted — and wrapped around, like a cocoon. After several firm requests for better behavior, I wound up gently and quietly bailing out on both of our behalves and driving our guest home. Mind you, the only way I was able to manage this was that, while Bruce was elsewhere, my mom was with us, and I could leave my two with her. If Grandma hadn't come along, we all would have had our outing severely abbreviated.

Then again, there will be times when "The Look" will be something that will utterly drop your jaw. I can recall one noteworthy evening when we had gone out for dinner. Ooh, new restaurant! New thrills, chills, and yes, let's not forget, spills to be had. One of those halfway houses that are elegant enough for the grown-ups, but still surprise you with menus the kids can color. This remarkable place furnished Elizabeth and Mikey each with a bag-o-crayons, AND a few teensy plastic dinosaurs to play with. The kids took full advantage, and then some.

As expected, some of the treats wound up on the floor, and we had a few rounds of low-volume whining and intramural arguing. I was frustrated, exhausted, and feeling guilty, so sure all I'd done, from soup to dessert, was scold. I wondered if maybe we should have just put on disguises at table and pretended we didn't notice anything. Then the people at the next table got up to leave (in a huff, I was sure), and the elder woman among them approached. Uh-oh! Those are always the self-appointed Emily Posts. She smiled at us and said "I just wanted to tell you how well-mannered your children are! They've been just lovely!"

Well, whaddya know?

Tips 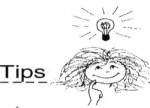 To Remember

✓ Your restaurant preferences will change — to kid-friendly places — with menus to color, child-pleasing meals, bright, colorful decor. And other families with children.

✓ This is NOT the time or place to entertain clients!

✓ Count on your kids to serve up a mishap or two while they're young. (Like spilling, dropping food and/or silverware, grabbing for the goodies on the table, ordering more than they can eat, losing their appetites, horning in on your dinner, delaying your dinner, interrupting your dinner, squirming in their seats, going exploring under the table, falling asleep in their plates, running and skipping (maybe INTO people), and getting carried away in the bathroom.)

✓ Sometimes, they MAY even eat.

✓ No matter what you do to avoid it, your child WILL have to take a bathroom break at the restaurant, and YOU will be the chosen escort. At least while he or she is young.

✓ You'll attract sympathy from SOME diners, and unwanted attention from others. You'll also be more patient with other active families also trying to get through dinner.

✓ Be prepared to take action. Maybe leaving before dinner arrives (be sure to leave some money behind to pay for the restaurant's troubles). Or ushering a loud little one outside until he or she calms down.

✓ Your child WILL become more manageable and cooperative — with time.

Chapter 10
Operation "Home Front"

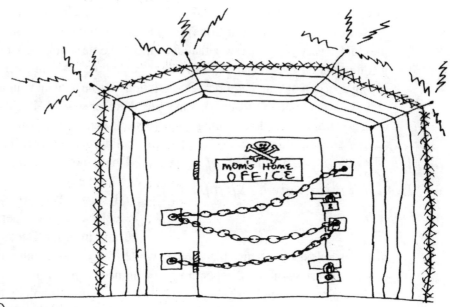

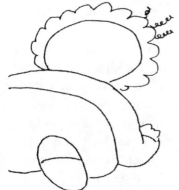

Many working moms have made a REALLY wonderful transition. Either they have a boss so enlightened or a job so user-friendly that they can actually move the whole works home. Or they're enterprising enough to have quit their job and started their own home-based business. This is an option that may become as irresistible to you as your new arrival is, and having tried it myself, I recommend it.

However you ought to think this through carefully! It is important that, at least while the child is very young, a few square feet in your home should be set aside, sacrosanct, just for your business. You MUST have a "cubbyhole" of your own. Even if it means giving up a part of your bedroom. One solution may be to evict your clothes from your only walk-in closet and set up shop in there. Another is to add hinges and a door to an ordinary alcove. Or add a heating unit and workspace to the garage or attic. Or even build yourself a shed in the back yard. (I have not yet completely ruled out a bomb shelter.)

You MUST have a "cubbyhole" of your own. Even if it means giving up a part of your bedroom.

If your little one isn't walking yet, you have a grace period to get your affairs in order. Because you can park him or her close by in a nice big playpen while you go about your business. Playpens come in a variety of sizes, depending on your needs and available space. And there are lots of mind-stimulating, safe, play-with-me objects to bolt on the sides. Things that will give your little one interesting things to think about and give you time to think, too.

However, my favorite device was a gift from my brother-in-law and his wife: a little wonder of a battery-powered swing-set with a form-fitted, padded seat that you can safely strap 'em into, and flick the switch. When the purring motor starts the rhythmic swinging, in a matter of moments, they're not only content as can be, they're flat-out asleep. And they're comfortable enough to be left as is for an hour or more. Mikey even appreciated its taste. This device only works to soothe the small-fry for a period of about six months. After that, when they're no longer confinable, you'd better have your home office security act together.

Regardless of their size, children have the vocal power of the Three Tenors combined. You'll need isolation from kid noise, if only for short periods, with a closed door and approved adult supervision on the other side. A small kid can "go off" like a smoke detector — a whole house full of them as a matter of fact — when you're on the phone trying to do business. Mine engage in tournament shouting, outsinging their favorite CD's, championship fire truck siren imitations, gas-passing simulations, and lately, squawking like Donald Duck. And sometimes it's not voices that present the problems.

At any given moment, I can expect to hear a piano, pots and pans, or Mikey's drum collection being pounded. Or his electric guitar — which he prefers to play Pete Townsend-style. There will be multiple series of stomps, clonks and thuds on the walls of any room in the house, probably because the kids are busy chasing or wrestling with each other — training to become human pinballs.

Or, since their grandparents gave each of them little battery-powered parrots with a recording mechanism that repeats the last half of your sentence back to you, I now hear them, times two. Especially Mikey, who seems to have been born with a megaphone in his mouth. His parrot sounds off on a regular basis, when one of us hasn't gutted it of its batteries, that is. Often there'll be "I can't find the Barbie car (Barbie car)!" squawking through the house. (And yes, it's Elizabeth's Barbie car, but the fact that it's a car means it's also Mikey's, once only slightly removed.) Occasionally, depending on where my son's parrot has followed him, it'll be "I can't come now, I'm makin' poo! (Makin' poo!)"

Needless to say, we make sure both parrots are electronically eviscerated when one of us is expecting a client to call or come by! Note this one mentally in big red letters.

No one ever thinks to anticipate this, let alone warn you about it. If your kid has any of those recording-talk-back toys, you MUST locate and disable them before you do business.

I'm thrilled that my little people are happy to have me within reach at a moment's notice when I'm conducting business at home. But I've had to work overtime to train them to respect my real need for quiet when I'm on the phone.

I may never live down the time I was discussing a new project involving Neil Young with a man at Warner Brothers Records. I figured — since I was safely hidden away in the privacy of my little home office — what difference could it make how I dressed? Or if I really hadn't "dressed" per se, since I got up? Well, there I was in the middle of my serious business call, when Mikey marched in, and gleefully trumpeted at the top of his four-year-old lungs, "Hey, Momma! I see your UNDER-WEAR!!!" I'm just grateful that I wasn't using the speaker-phone!

It's not only your professional image you'll still be striving to protect and maintain. Your papers, files, and office supplies are vulnerable to being chewed on, barfed on, scribbled on, crawled over, wadded up, used as a placemat, or walked off with, the moment your attention is elsewhere.

One example occurred late one evening. We were scanning small objects for a catalogue project when we reached for a ruler for a sizing reference. It was there a minute ago, wasn't it? Well, nice try. All of our grown-up-style rulers had mysteriously disappeared. Our kids had apparently decided they liked ours better than theirs and set up their own exchange program. Leaving my husband in a foul mood, and offering his kingdom for "a ruler that doesn't have Garfield on it." Moments later, he was grabbing for his car keys to make yet another inconvenient trip to the 24-hour convenience store.

You MUST provide sanctuary — where your rolodex won't be doodled on, rifled through, or rearranged. Elizabeth thoughtfully re-ordered mine one day, after being inspired to reinvent the alphabet. Protect your work — so new illustrations and coded messages won't mysteriously appear in the pages of your appointment book, invoices or business stationery. Or so none of those will be snipped into with a pair of kiddy scissors. Beware, for your diaries could easily end up as doilies.

Your stapler risks being rediscovered as a musical instrument: the perfect Ka-CHUNKing device. We all REALLY know how much fun this is. Then you'll find an empty stapler and a layer of Ka-CHUNK'ed staples now covering your office floor. This, incidentally, will happen at the precise moment you need to staple a presentation together before dashing off to a meeting you're already late for. When you've just smoothed on your nice new stockings, but haven't yet slipped into your shoes.

You MUST defend your desk from being finger-painted. Make sure it can't be overrun with pre-school art projects, doll tea parties, coloring books, or an entire miniature fire station. Or lunch!

Shelter your work chair from greasy, sticky fingerprints or mud from the backyard. Or else — you may get the news only after you sit down. Or maybe it's the valued client you're entertaining who'll be the first to know.

Safeguard your phone where it won't be commandeered, slobbered into, fiddled with, or deprogrammed. Where unrecognizable numbers won't turn up on your phone bill. One afternoon, at the ripe old age of 16 months, Mikey called Baltimore. Make sure you secure the telephone where the receiver can't be mysteriously cocked JUST off the hook — leaving you waiting for clients to call you back and wondering why there's been no action all day?

And let's not forget that never-ending crusade to keep your computer SAFE! Ah, here's a good one I'll borrow from my husband, who has spent his share of time as a working "Mr. Mom" himself.

He's a computer consultant, headquartered at home. And he's learned the hard way, as have I to a lesser degree, to protect his computer. Mikey wandered into Bruce's office one day and, with a few impressive, although random, key strokes, managed to rename one of Bruce's main computer files. What for ages had been a familiar name had magically turned into "mft225tt." It cost him precious business time figuring out what was suddenly wrong with the computer, and then correcting it.

And then there was the time we were trying to copy a very important file from a disk. Seems simple enough, right? Just pop that little diskette into the disk drive, hit the right keys and zip, it's done. But in this case, it wasn't zip; it was a resounding GRIND! Neither of us could determine why the floppy drive and the hard drive were no longer on speaking terms. Until something slightly sickening dawned on us.

Do you remember the TV commercial awhile back that showed a daddy coaxing his toddler to eat his oatmeal? "This is how we feed our hungry baby, my son." A few moments later, Junior gets the bright idea that the VCR is hungry and "feeds" it some oatmeal, too. We once thought this commercial was hilarious. Until we became parents, that is, and experienced our own personalized version of it.

We suddenly realized OUR son had decided the computer must be simply starving for little round cardboard "pogs." He made sure that the computer's floppy drive had a full meal of them. What resulted was beyond merely severe computer indigestion. Jamming all those pogs into that little slot gave the floppy drive a case of permanent illiteracy. Another loss of valuable business time, a business tool, and fifty bucks to have the messed-up component replaced.

A computer mishap can result from something ridiculously simple. The mere act of one of the kids trying to cozy up with us has been a flirtation with disaster.

If she spies me sitting down, wherever it may be, Elizabeth loves to sneak up beside me, snake one of her legs up over my lap and pull the rest of herself up after it. Or climb on top of me from the back. But at times, I've been at my desk, furiously editing away on some writing assignment and find this display a little, well, inconvenient. She can jostle my arm while I'm moving a block of text JUST enough to send the entire block off to Never-Never Land.

And I'm always afraid of having them bump the computer, or the table it's on, throwing it out of whack in some way. Computers, modems, disk drives, and the like are NOT built to be shaken or stirred, are they?

And while I crave close, physical interplay with both my kids, the smallest interruption can completely derail my train of thought. Not to mention how completely scummy and traitor-ish I feel because I may have to spurn their affections, even if only momentarily.

While he or she is very young, a kid will regard any computer as downright irresistible. SO much fun to touch. Covered with buttons of every imaginable kind. Some cute little lights here and there that wink at you. A big screen up there at eye view — ahh! Another TV! Sometimes its disk drive makes pleasant little purring noises. "New kitty in there, Mommy?" It'll be the best toy they've ever seen, other than the big cardboard box it came in.

They've just GOTTA touch it. And they do. They WILL find a way. Or die trying. And until they can be cyber-weaned, they don't know their own strength. Just as each of my tiny tots could tromp through the house with the footsteps of a circus elephant, so, too, with their fingers. They wouldn't just try to push the buttons on the keyboard. They'd press and punch and pound. Their little index fingers become miniature jackhammers. And if they can get the computer to bleep in protest, so much the better.

And, all of this compounds when it comes to your laptop, which is portable — something that can be dragged around. Sat upon. Danced on. Or driven over.

Then again, there's that whole set of potential misadventures with the Internet . . .

Neither of my children has yet figured out how to gain access, thank heavens! The computer they CAN get to, the old spare where we put their drawing and town-building programs, and reading and math games, isn't linked up on-line anywhere. And for now, we're both savoring the breathing room we have while they're still young and don't care about such things — yet.

Now here's something else I'm positive you won't have anticipated. No one does (unless they're VERY computer-savvy). And it's only by having a cyber-nerd of a husband with years of cold, hard experience that I found this out: You wanna see a computer mishap? Consider the risk to your software from a wandering refrigerator magnet that just hitched a ride inside an innocent little hand, and landed a little too close by. Or a piece of those darling little wooden train sets that are so beautifully simple in their design, and link up, car-to-car, by magnetic ends.

Magnets can be profoundly toxic to computers. Magnets can lobotomize computers. Because they erase the electronic information within. Same thing can happen when a magnet meets recording tape. That means if audio or video cassettes matter at all to your business affairs, from phone machine message cassettes to any tape library system you may have assembled, you'd BETTER take precautions. And be downright ferocious about it, too. Bruce also notes that while distance and strength do play a part, one should keep magnets away from computers. That's why there are no magnets in our office.

Kids love office supplies. Things like your mailing tubes and stamps, neat padded envelopes, and that bubble-wrap stuff (deliriously enticing, and noisy), glue sticks, post-it pads, markers (the more colorful, the better), checks, invoices, customer records, file-folders, all are just begging to be toyed with, or spirited away.

My husband has learned to keep what he calls his "100-dollar tape dispenser" practically under lock and key. Bruce became thoroughly frustrated one afternoon when he couldn't find his office tape dispenser for something like the 94th time. The same one he'd replaced on multiple occasions. Well, this was the absolute last straw! So he stormed off to the nearest office supply store and stocked up, something fierce, on tape dispensers. About a hundred dollars' worth, as it turned out. By the time the kids have found, and "borrowed" all but the last one, he figures, that single survivor will win the official title: "the 100-dollar tape dispenser."

Mikey nearly gave us both heart failure not long ago, after he spotted our industrial-size packing-tape dispenser. Simply HAD to finger it. Just a little. Problem was, not only did it have wickedly sharp, flesh-eating points on its tape-tearing edge, but also, it was sitting on a paper-cutter, high up, out of view on what we thought was a too-high-for-kids shelf. So we stood the chance of a multiple-choice trip to the hospital. How any of us survived THAT episode, I'm still trying to figure out. No less, how Mikey knew to climb that high, and specifically to that spot on that shelf at that end of the room.

Oopsies of many kinds are just a breath, or a wiggle, away. Consider the rolling office chair. It can roll right over little toes if your kid comes in, feeling cuddly, and steps up too close while your concentration is elsewhere. Same thing could afflict little fingers as they slither around underfoot. The high shelves full of heavy books, manuals, or tools? An avalanche just panting to be set off. A desk lamp that's been on for awhile means there's potential for burns. Any electrical cords and cables, no matter how out-of-reach you may think they are, can be tripped over or otherwise goofed with. The paper-cutter I just mentioned? I don't even want to think about it.

And obviously, ANY work that relies on serious tools or chemicals needs to be strictly and meticulously confined. In my case, much of that involves all my pliers and other jewelers' tools, the tissue-slicing blades, hole pokers, and the pasta machine for my polymer clay work. And all that irresistible silver and gold fill wire! Ooo, yummy! Sure beats pipe cleaners, doesn't it?

You HAVE to be able to lock yourself and your home business in. If your little one can get to you, you'll wind up paying for it.

Believe me, it's all isolated, and even though I do plenty of art and craft work with both Elizabeth and Mikey, neither of them gets near any of it without a chaperone.

You HAVE to be able to lock yourself and your home business in. If your little one can get to you, and trust me, it's usually right when you're intensely involved in some serious wheeling and dealing, you'll wind up paying for it. Like the time Mikey walked in on Bruce while he was working with the mouse. Mikey grabs Daddy's arm (of course, the one with the mouse on the end), and jostles him good. It happens so quickly that Daddy isn't able to stop the computer from moving several important files to another location. Which means those files are effectively lost for awhile, as is still more precious business time while we search the system for them. However, I'm told it could have been worse. They could just as easily have been deleted.

Frequently, we find ourselves parroting one of Mikey's more recent favorite phrases: "Guess we gotta get a new one!" Believe me, all it takes — whether you're in or out on some errand — is one good wrestling match, tug-o-war, relay race, balloon toss, go-fetch, chase-the-cat, ride-the-dog, or argument between siblings or your kid and a visiting friend, and your elaborate and costly computer set-up is on its side, on the floor, in pieces.

At times, even something so small as one little finger in the wrong place, is enough to initiate a disaster. Mikey's little finger, for one, is more powerful than a locomotive and is able to leap tall barricades in a single bound.

I was in the process of printing out a critically-important business letter to Tim Allen on our expensive new color printer. You know how it is — where the letterhead on the stationery must look incontrovertibly pristine, and the presentation has to be just so. Everything was humming along fine until almost the end — when I heard this crackle-crackle-CRUNCH! Seems the finished letter was being fed out, right into a big, folded-up newspaper that neither of US had left there, precisely in the way of the printer's feeder tray. The letter got jammed, big time — and naturally, in exactly the worst way for the printer's inner workings.

Then I remembered that Mikey had visited, only minutes beforehand, squeezing in between my chair and the desk with the printer on it. With one deft little motion, he'd flicked that newspaper aside — right into the path of the outflowing printer paper — to make more room for himself. Then he'd left. And so did our printer, as it turns out, until we could get it fixed. I never had the nerve to explain to Tim Allen's representative the REAL reason why I was late on that one!

There's another reason why you need secure surroundings in which to do business. Every so often, you'll HAVE to have some uninterrupted time to complete a project, an extended phone call, a presentation, a print-out, or whatever. I guarantee that if you take a moment out for a breather, and poke your wary head outside your office door for even an instant, the very whiff of you will alert your little one like red meat to a football player, and BING! You're officially busted. You will then break your mood, concentration, and the corresponding distraction of your kid toward something other than you.

And about the same time, I promise you, you'll probably be waiting on "hold," in the middle of a phone call with your vacationing accountant's assistant who is trying to track down a check that was supposed to have arrived a couple of days ago. Then your mom will call on the other line, then the doorbell will ring with a neighborhood kid asking to play with yours.

We've had moments when multiples of activities magically coincided with the tea kettle going off, the toast burning (because I hadn't realized it was on a setting that would keep toasting), the spin cycle on the washing machine suddenly spinning madly out of balance and out of control, and the cat jumping up into the tuna salad the kids hadn't finished eating an hour ago. And sometimes, when I was still working at the AP and thought I was finished for the day, my beeper would go off, and it would be Washington needing something RIGHT NOW!

What is really being said here is that it is much harder to focus on your job while juggling a kid at home.

What is really being said here is that it is much harder to focus on your job while juggling a kid at home. ESPECIALLY when he or she does, like my Mikey, who wants to break in with some statement like, "Mom, I need to give you a kiss right now." And my resolve immediately liquefies and I have to shout, "Stop the presses!" It never fails. And besides, you can't even reasonably get mad about an interruption like that!

I recommend your office setup be situated close to a bathroom, a workable window or door to the outside if you're in need of a smoke break, and a portable coffee maker. In my case, it's a microwave oven in which I heat up one of my hundreds of cups of tea in any given day. If you have to cross the house to get to the kitchen for something, or the bathroom's in the next county, you're bound to be intercepted.

I often found myself reheating the same cup of tea nine or ten different times before I took this advice to heart. I'd start one. Then I'd get distracted on the way back to my office by a little one needing me for something. If I was lucky enough both to solve the problem AND to return to my project, I'd forget about my cup of tea in the process. And by the time I remembered it, my drink would be cold and I'd have to start the process all over again. And I'd have to cross back through THEIR territory to do so.

One small consolation to that episode: I now almost always know precisely where to hunt for my tea cup whenever I realize it's unaccounted for.

Just as you need to lock yourself in, you have an equally pressing need to lock that office door behind you whenever you leave, even if it's just for a few minutes. And while you're at it, start stashing away some spare money in your business account for the inevitable equipment repairs!

Get ready to juggle house-calls. Not the ones some kindly doctors used to make. The ones you may become responsible for, especially if your business involves consulting, or in my husband's case, troubleshooting somebody else's computer — on THEIR turf.

On the other hand, the client may have to come to you, as sometimes happens to me, to look at the newest beads, jewelry, or artwork I've designed. In this case, it's usually better to set up a rendezvous in neutral territory.

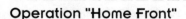

No matter how carefully you arrange meetings away from home, there WILL be occasions when colleagues will have to come to you. That's when you'll have to be able to shove stray toys, sneakers, and science experiments under the closest available dust ruffle, set up a good play place, project, special video, or other well-earned distraction for the little people, and THEN go to it.

And CHECK THE BATHROOM. Some little person you love may have just visited the commode and forgotten to flush!

Then again, one fine day you might be surprised to find that you suddenly have a lovely assistant eager to stand by that box on the display floor. As Elizabeth grows older, she's become more interested in the art and design side of my home business, and she is eager to be my helper. She's actually run to the kitchen to bring our guests a glass of ice water, or shown them the way to the bathroom while I have to go fumble for something. I find her little voice piping up from time to time, proudly throwing her two cents in about a new design of mine, almost as though she's my agent. As he comes along behind her, Mikey is startling me with some of the same participation.

In this case, make sure you have something treat-worthy with which to reward any little helpers in your life, after your guest leaves. We'll both always be glad we discovered the wonderful world of "Treasure Tickets." Encourage your children to cooperate by having them earn tickets for good behavior. Keep an envelope with their name on it, maybe scribbled or decorated by them. When they get ten treasure tickets, they win the right to go to the treasure box and select a present. None of these "treasures" needs to be more than a dollar or two each, so you won't have to look farther than the nearest well-stocked drug store for good kid-loot.

Advantage one: They learn to earn things, particularly if they're too young for an actual allowance. Advantage two: They find out about saving up for various reasons and that gratification isn't always instantaneous. Advantage three: They learn to count. Advantage four: They have good reason to get with the program of YOUR choice.

Another great way to motivate your kid to do your bidding when he or she would rather have it the other way is: to encourage a controlled amount of misbehavior as a trade-off. Here's a neat one: When you tell offspring it won't be possible for them to sit in on the meeting with you, or visit with the client you and your kid both know well (or, for that matter, ANY topic on your agenda towards which they might be contrary), your child's first reaction will be to protest verbally. That's good. And you should say so. I'm not kidding.

Around our house it goes like this: "OK, you're both going to have to blah-blah-blah (some behavior the kids do NOT want to have to do), and I'd like a medium amount of whining, please." And boy, do they fall all over themselves to obey THAT order! Then, you say, "OK, now I need a LARGE amount of whining, please." Again, you'll be astounded at the level of compliance. Then, you say, "OK, now may I have NO whining, please." And, amazingly enough, they're right with you then, too. Of course, by that time, it's become a game, and a joke, and you've kidded them out of their pigheadedness while allowing them to have their mad-on in complete safety. Strange but true.

Depending on the client and the activity, I find it can actually be an enhancement to have the kids close by. If you luck into a client with one or more kids the same age as yours, celebrate that! They can all go play together in one room or outside, while you have your meeting with their parental unit. As they get older and have observed you in action, they'll be able to judge for themselves when to assist and when to make themselves scarce.

Mary Steenburgen once told me this worked out more than beautifully for her while she was filming the movie *Parenthood*. As many actresses (especially those with clout) now do, she'd brought her two kids on location with her. Perhaps it was the nature of this particular film, but "Parenthood" turned out to be the prevailing theme off the set as well as on. Seems everybody else of the parent persuasion, from director Ron Howard on down, had brought his or her kids along, and all the little people wound up happily running around and playing together for weeks.

In a unique case such as this, you may actually build a more solid relationship with your client because you both have kid-pals in common, which isn't bad for business. For all you know, the person you're dealing with may be having one of those days with a too-full schedule and no place to park the little one. And man, will they appreciate you! But, again, DON'T assume this is true with any client until you get to know them well.

Expect some conflicts as you move through this stage. They'll be inevitable.

One case for me was an occasion that sounded too good to be true — an opportunity to mix work and kids that was actually fun and productive for everybody all around. We got an invitation to an industry screening of *The Flintstones*. A family screening, on a Saturday morning, and all the show-biz types from cast to crew to critics could cover the film, make the scene, schmooze and do business, and you were SUPPOSED to bring the kids. And that, we did.

Only Mikey got a little carried away. He was young enough to be discovering his language skills. Mikey has always functioned on two gears: full-throttle-top-of-his-lungs and out-cold-asleep. Naturally, this occasion was not one of the snoozers. We were about 45 minutes into the movie, in a packed theater, when Mikey began to sound off. "GO — GET — DADDY'S — CAR!" "GO — SEE — CAR!" "LET'S — GO — HOME!" "I — WANT — DADDY'S — CAR!" Even John Goodman's loudest Fred Flintstone bombast in widescreen Dolby and THX theater sound processing was no match for my son. Needless to say we had to scoop up everyone, everyone's *Flintstones* party favors AND all our portable baby gear, and get out of there before we alienated half of Hollywood.

Elizabeth once got very upset with me, in the middle of a visit with some colleagues who'd become clients. Trust me, she'd already been told clearly, in detail, and in advance, that this was business — even though she'd met these people multiple times before. Regardless, she still decided they were simply company coming over, and WHY COULDN'T SHE TAKE HER TURN WITH THEM? AND SHOW THEM ALL HER BARBIE MAGAZINES?! Mikey then got on the bandwagon (that happens a lot when there's more than one. You automatically have to multiply any behavior exhibitions by the number of small-fry present), and wanted equal time to show off his newest toy cars.

If it's a client you know well or have dealt with for quite awhile, the pressure's off somewhat. They'll already know you and your circumstances, and it's likely they'll understand. But still, you'll prefer to be undistracted. New clients? Go alone to their place. Or take them out for coffee, or to a restaurant or juice bar somewhere. It's usually much easier to hold your meetings in the field.

As my little people get older, I've discovered that there are a few other unexpected disadvantages that you have to work past, assuming, of course, that you want to exude a professional image while conducting your business at home. They will tend to want to race you to the phone and to the doorbell, no matter what they may have to interrupt. Eating. Playing. Hanging out with their best friend who's come over for further adventures with Barbie or Spiderman. Certainly, doing homework.

I really have to lean on them to stay with what they're doing and not to bolt away. You never want them running out and simply flinging open the door just because the bell rang. Child protection concerns take over here. And if it's a client, YOU want to be answering that door and keeping control of the situation. Besides, Mikey can't always be guaranteed to be fully dressed at any given moment.

You also do NOT want them tying up the phone with their pals as they get older. And tie up the phone they will. Jane Withers once advised me that as soon as her kids were big enough, she started deducting pre-set amounts from their allowances depending on how long they spent on the phone. She says they wised up quickly.

Another phenomenon I've found comes into play as the kids grow older involves their exercise of imaginative language skills.

At any rate, you should still set aside your own number for your business, and do it now. Our needs compelled us to install a whole network of them. Another separate line for the fax-modem. Still another one or two strictly for on-line purposes.

Think through carefully what your own logistics are as to whether you want to restrict where your business phone rings. You may have it so organized that it should ring ONLY in your office. No temptation to anybody else in the house that way. But, if your business calls tend to happen in spurts, here and there, throughout the day, during which you may be doing any number of other things all around the house, you may have to let your business line ring in additional rooms. It helps to have a phone with a hold button, if you're in the kitchen when your call comes, and you really need to be at your desk to deal with it. And every phone in our house does have speakerphone capability.

Another phenomenon I've found comes into play as the kids grow older involves their exercise of imaginative language skills — and of your sense of humor — depending on what state of wear-down it's in at any given moment.

My two decided it was the most hilarious thing on earth to start spouting out such edifying verbiage as "Poo-poo! Pee-pee! Stinky-yucky-trash!! Fart!!!" Sometimes spoken, sometimes sung. Frequently accented with sound effects. Some of them RATHER authentic. Almost always at full volume. Followed by spasms of giggles that can last for several minutes apiece. As it was one fine day when I was trying to set up an interview with John Travolta (who can probably relate anyway, though, since he is a dad). And it can become like "Dueling Banjos" as they go back and forth goading each other onward and downward, circling the drain as it were, trying to top each other with wilder and weirder permutations.

It can go on all day long. In our case, it has been darn near continuous for a couple of years. Well, that might be tolerable on occasion, depending on how freewheeling your mood is, or when you all are at home and at play. But when you're in business mode and trying to work it's absolutely the pits. This is another one of those moments when you DON'T want to be on speakerphone. You may at times

You MUST prevent their mixing phone addictions with language arts.

wish you were back in that old office building you left behind. It does not enhance your professional image one bit, when you clap your hand over the mouthpiece and hiss at the kids to be quiet because you're in the middle of a phone call.

You MUST prevent their mixing phone addictions with language arts like these. Imagine the consternation of a friend of mine whose daughter KNEW it was her best friend calling her one fateful afternoon. Phone rings. Girl gets there first. Picks it up and merrily hollers "Hello, Fart-Face!" into the mouthpiece. You know what happened next, don't you? The voice on the other end of the line wasn't the girl's best friend, but her mom's best prospect — who HAD been about to close a lucrative deal with her.

I'm hopeful that I've already taken sufficient precautions against this one happening to me. Having my own separate business line does help. But it still gets a little unhinged around our house every so often. Thank heavens none of those instances so far has coincided with a visit from a client. Because from time to time, and without advance warning my little ones love to race around the house without a stitch on. It can be at somewhat understandable moments when they've just climbed out of the bathtub and they're feeling so frisky that you have to darn near tackle 'em to get their clothes put on. At other times, it's simply when the mood strikes.

Mikey, in particular, takes delight in doing this. Moreover, he may decide to indulge in, shall we say, self-discovery, fairly frequently once he's liberated himself from the stifling shackles of jeans, T-shirts, and underwear. Just the thing to put the finishing touch on that ol' professional image of yours when a vision like that charges by.

I'm grateful they only pull this stunt when they're most comfortable, and only their Daddy and I are at home and not entertaining clients! So far, this has only infringed upon my business dealings when I've been on the phone. But I've still been forced to shut my office door against the noise and commotion of one of those spur-of-the-moment skin stampedes. Because our version of *Rawhide* is every bit as loud as it is eye-popping.

Tips 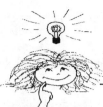 To Remember

✓ You may decide to move your job or business home to be closer to your child. Therefore, you MUST be smart about your home office.

✓ You will need a special area or room that's SET ASIDE, AND SECURE, just for your business, so you can work in safety and peace without interruption.

✓ You should be able to isolate yourself in it, even if only for short periods. It should include, or be near, a bathroom and a coffee or tea maker. You can remain isolated for awhile, that way.

✓ While your child is young, he or she is more easily confinable — in playpens and other baby accessories.

✓ But when he or she is no longer confinable: Make sure you have approved adult supervision when YOU can't watch your child. You should be able to escape (at least partially) from the kid-noise — either from their mouths or their toys. Beware talking toys, especially.

✓ Make sure your office, office supplies, business phones, desk and work chair, your phone and phone lines, AND your computer are protected from the young, curious, and adventuresome. (Your computer is particularly tempting.)

✓ No magnets! They're bad for computers, VHS tapes, and audio cassettes.

✓ One of many reasons to keep kids out: You'll need blocks of time to work. Many of your office tools and supplies, including paper-cutters, staples, shelves with heavy contents, electrical cords, chemicals, electrical wires can pose a danger to a child. Much of your office equipment is vulnerable and expensive to replace and repair.

- ✓ Better save up for those expenses, anyway! Your child is more clever than you know!

- ✓ All is not totally lost if you are home with your child while you have to do business.

- ✓ If a client is coming to you, check the bathroom first — in case your kid's forgotten to flush.

- ✓ Your kid may want to participate or assist in your meetings. This is possible only: When your child is older and more responsible. To go get your guest a drink or show him or her to the bathroom. Or when your client is an equally frazzled working parent, with his or her own kid in tow. Yours can entertain the little visitor. This works well only if you know the client well.

- ✓ Any good behavior must be reinforced!

- ✓ Try the "treasure ticket" reward system.

- ✓ Allow a CONTROLLED AMOUNT of misbehavior or whining as a trade-off.

- ✓ A kid at home may want to race you to the front door or the phone — which you DO NOT want. Discourage him or her from tying up the phone.

- ✓ Set up your own phone line exclusively for business.

- ✓ Figure out what modifications it needs (where do you want it to ring, do you need one with speakerphone or intercom capability)?

- ✓ Be aware of your child's urges to fire off some "wild" language on the phone or in the background.

- ✓ Be aware of your child's urges to run around in various stages of undress. This can happen during your business call OR your client's visit.

Chapter 11
Entertaining The Troops

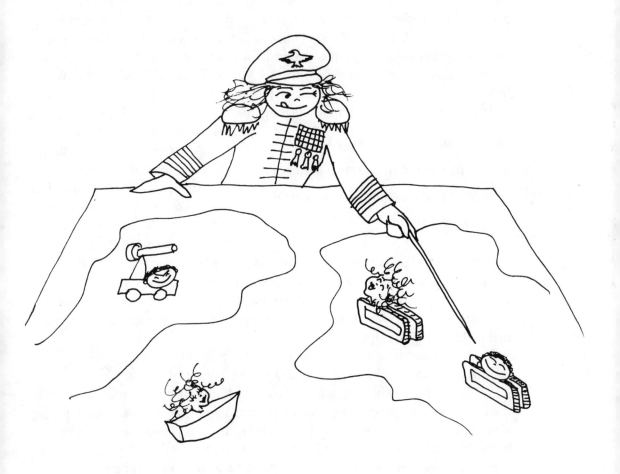

In one respect, when you're juggling job and Junior, you really can have it all. Maybe not all the time — it's best to have a separate room for your business. You'll need to have plans and coordination like an army general but it's definitely workable.

The best solution I've found when I need to do business and the little ones are home with me includes options that relocate the children. Such as: a visit to Grandma or another close relative for a few hours. A playday with a neighborhood friend, or a close pal from school. A drop-off for story-time at the local library. My husband has even taken the children along with him on errands or other brief car rides.

Often, though, arranging a field trip for your child is not a possibility. With a little thinking and planning, you can safely station the little one elsewhere in or around your home with an intriguing assignment that he or she will be eager to do.

If it's a nice day outside you may wish to set up a project in the backyard that's messy enough to keep him or her engrossed, and, even better, "grossed out."

This is the time to open that new, deluxe box of crayons with the 197,000 colors in it. Better yet, throw in a post-it pad or two. This affords them not only something to color on, but also something they can proudly hang up on the wall in an instant. You'll discover soon enough that there's no such thing as too many crayons. Thankfully, they're not expensive, and I try to keep several extras hidden away for such purposes. Same thing with new coloring books, books in general, stencil sets, puzzles. A nice new Matchbox racer or car road map will never fail to make Mikey mighty happy.

If it's a nice day outside you may wish to set up a project in the backyard that's messy enough to keep him or her engrossed, and, even better, "grossed out," for awhile.

Such enticing activities include mud cooking (mud wrestling would be more like it with my two), finger-painting, bug collecting, digging for worms, or bowl licking if you just finished making frosting for a cake. You could even turn the cake over to the kid and have him or her frost it. Or if you have other plans for the cake, surrender a load of cookies or doughnuts to be iced. Your child can design and execute an entire custom picnic if you merely provide the right components. If it's a really hot day, leave them alone with the rest of the ice cream container and a big spoon. You won't hear a peep out of your munchkin for quite some time with that one!

You have to think of something relatively safe, with blunt edges (And no swimming pool or balcony), that doesn't involve constant adult supervision. Sidewalk chalk and washable paints are also excellent for this, provided the pavement is somewhere safe. Have them decorate some old flower pots for you. Or a piece of sacrificial lawn furniture or a garden fixture. We have a sacrificial lawn, as a matter of fact. One fine day Bruce and I threw up our hands together and decided to relinquish control of the backyard to them, for a few years. They littered the place with their push toys, trikes, bikes, wagons, kiddy cars, and other stuff. We handed over old pots and pans, bent spoons, and dishwasher-warped plastic containers, with and without lids. Same thing for bats and balls of all sizes, hula hoops, jump ropes, and anything else we could think of. And plastic everything.

One fine day Bruce and I threw up our hands and decided to relinquish control of the backyard to them.

Our backyard started to look like a disatster area. We even had a freeway back there for awhile, where they wore away the grass with their assorted racing activities. Pits, too, and not just for pit stops. They had to quarry their own mud for their mud cuisine, don't you know? We decided to let them have their fun back there and not sweat it 'til they'd grown out of it. By then, we reasoned, we could reseed the back yard with new grass and scrape the remaining paint smears off the patio. In the meantime, though, this scheme has repeatedly yielded two well-occupied, creatively-stimulated, and extremely dirty children. Hey, no big deal! You can always hose 'em down or plop 'em in the bathtub when you come back up for air and want them to come back in. They can even paint the hose if they feel so inclined.

Once an offspring grows a little older, award him or her with the hose, for work AND play purposes. When it came to the garden hose, my kids had to be closely supervised when they were young. If Mikey had had his way, our entire backyard would have become a pool, and probably the entire neighborhood, too. We almost had to take the handle off the pipe it was connected to, in order to keep him from it. Soon, though, Elizabeth was old enough to play Big Sister and supervise him, and scold him by proxy for me. (Boy, is THAT ever a delicious assignment for an older sibling!) And before we knew it, they were both old enough to play responsibly with the hose, AND water the garden properly.

But what if bad weather conditions or other circumstances force you to be shut-ins? Indoors, where you'd probably like to keep it cleaner overall, I've found that our home movies pay some very nice residuals.

The arrival of any little one in your life will probably be accompanied by the arrival of a video camera, if you don't have one already. We have a rapidly expanding library of home videos, all featuring our kids in choice moments around home, on vacation, at school events, and beyond. Pull out a movie starring offspring, hit the play button, microwave some popcorn or unwrap the graham crackers or another age-appropriate treat, and let him or her luxuriate. Your kid is guaranteed to find the subject matter fascinating for a generous chunk of time, and you'll get a breather to go do some business. Besides, your conscience won't be quite so guilt-ridden about plopping the little one in front of the TV in a case like this.

Oh yes, and don't be afraid to use a little neighborly kindness to its greatest advantage. Any activity that you can park your kid next to, for an hour or so, in safety and comfort, you can just as easily park a friend's or neighbor's kid, too. This strategy can yield several dividends.

First, whole new kingdoms-to-be-conquered can open up when a friend comes over. Sometimes they'll float along with the prevailing current you stirred up. At other times, they'll become distracted by one another, and will probably leave your idea behind for one or more of their own making. It's come to the point around our house where, if Elizabeth's "honorary sister" Tessie comes over from next door, or Chris, Mikey's best buddy from preschool, is here, all the kids start playing together and taking care of themselves.

Second, if it's something really creative that you've thought up for them to do, and they're really into it, perhaps you've set off a spark within the mind of your little visitor.

Third, you automatically endear yourself to the little visitor's mom, who will greatly appreciate that you gave her a respite. You gain yourself an ally, and someone with whom to reciprocate. The fellow-frazzled working mom you help today will be glad to return the favor when you're in some carnivorous boss-activated or assignment-activated bind. Do this with more than one such mom and you multiply your own future options accordingly.

Here's one of my absolute favorite ways for distracting kids long enough for you to get a few things done:

You know all those brown paper bags you get with every trip to the grocery store? I keep stashing them in a kitchen corner, feeling too guilty about throwing them out, and reusing them more slowly than they accumulate. Now, every so often I take a dozen of them or so (the more the better) and rip 'em all up into little pieces, about three to six inches each. Then I throw all those little pieces on the floor in the middle of the living room.

The kids are drawn to this drift of urban "leaves" like flies to cowpies. They jump into them, throw them around, scoop them up, roll in them, bury each other in them, stomp around and squeal a lot. They may continue to do this for at least a half-hour at a time. And after they run off to do something else, they return almost slavishly to repeat those procedures and invent new ones. At the end of the day, you just "rake" up the leaves with your fingers, and leave them in a nice neat pile in a corner of the room.

And/or have the kids help you do so. They'll find the pile and make very good use of it again tomorrow, I promise you. And the day after tomorrow. And on from there.

I found that it suited my schedule not to retire the pile for maybe a week or two. One time I let it go for more than a month. They loved it. Their friends loved it. Elizabeth's kindergarten party go-ers adored it. More, even, than they did the professionally-organized kid activities we'd paid for in the back yard! The only real dilemma you'll have is whether to surprise them with it, or have them help you make it in the first place. That, alone, is an activity worth its weight in gold, because how often is a kid actually encouraged to rip something up into shreds?

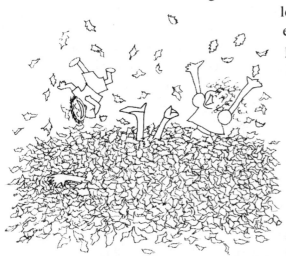

Grown-ups coming over? Well, move it, or have your child help you move it, to his or her room. You might even just build it all there and keep it there if the adults who'll be visiting happen to be business clients. If not, and they've got young kids of their own, don't sweat it. Go right ahead and leave it in the living room. They won't view it as a mess you're too lazy to clean up. They'll recognize it as an award-winning kid entertainment, and they'll think you're brilliant. You may find one or more moms or dads climbing in with their kids to test-drive it for themselves. And you're liable to see the same mess alive and kicking all over THEIR living room floors the next time you go visit them.

While that mess is easy to live with, I've found others that are nearly impossible, and these seem to pop up at the most inopportune moments — like when you're all dressed and JUST about to leave for a meeting. It usually comes with a vacuum cleaner and a spray bottle of Windex (or something similar) surgically attached. And it's positively guaranteed to be something you never planned for or were warned about!

Remember all those mysterious spots and stickies I mentioned awhile back? The stickies especially. They're almost always sweet. Which means what you REALLY have are mysterious little beacons being beamed directly into the nearest ant colony.

It happened to me on the way out to a Kevin Costner interview — a rare one-on-one I'd FINALLY snagged after months of begging and coaxing and cajoling, and had to give up part of a rainy Saturday for. I was literally zooming for the front door when what to my wondering eyes did appear, but a miniature army with eight THOUSAND tiny soldiers in it. They'd been flooded out of their ant colony just outside the back door and were now laying siege to one of those little sticky spots on our family room rug.

You can throw your hands up and continue toward the front door and hope the swarm won't overrun the whole house by the time you get back, or do a quick 'n dirty fix-it job to stanch the flow. There was enough of them that I felt compelled to do SOMETHING quick, because I was SURE some young 'un would find reason to rummage around in them if I didn't take at least SOME corrective action. What I felt driven to do because I'd built in a grace period beforehand (PLAN-NING! I MEAN IT! IT'LL SAVE YOUR SKIN!) was to grab the vacuum for the first infantry unit and spritz with Windex to discourage the second. It works just as well as the poison bug spray you might resort to if kids weren't on the battlefield, too.

It takes a good five to ten extra minutes, plus a few more for you to calm down and tuck your shirt tails back in. In my case, it cost me the first half of a general press session with Costner that I'd planned to catch ALL of, for backstopping purposes, before I went in for my private interview with him. That was OK. That was optional anyway. Once we were underway,

Costner gave me a strange look from time to time. It wasn't just my probing questions. It was my fidgeting every so often, because I was certain there were leftover ants crawling up my legs.

Stick the following to your brain like so much bubble gum to a carpet, especially if you are accustomed to a clean, well-ordered world: A KID IS A CRUMB-DROP-PER. Crumbs of everything. Crumbs from stuff that you wouldn't think would even HAVE crumbs! They will rain down crumbs of all kinds all over the place, step on 'em, and then track 'em every place else. And you will, too, before you realize it. They WILL wind up inside your office sanctuary even if you somehow manage to keep the little one out of there all the time. I've found that with or without household help, I've had to vacuum almost on a daily basis. And not just to keep visiting clients from being totally grossed-out. It's simply so we can stand it, ourselves!

Sometimes messes can be your friend, as I pointed out earlier. The trick is to CONTAIN and CONTROL them.

I've also found that a sure-fire way to locate virtually any mess such as dried pudding blobs on the dining room chairs, or crayon marks on the walls, is during a narrow window of time that starts about a minute before the doorbell rings with your client or another VIP. It ends somewhere in the midst of your meeting.

You'll become quite deft at nudging toys, stray kid spoons, and half-eaten cookies behind doors and under furniture. I've even moved large portions of the living room around to hide something at the last minute. If your home has any large potted plants, decorator gourds, pillows, footstools, or other artifacts that accent corners, these are good quick 'n dirty concealers, too. Provided, of course, that your child hasn't stealthily hung some used underwear on it.

Sometimes messes can be your friend, as I pointed out earlier. The trick is to CONTAIN and CONTROL them. There's a simple way to corral an inside mess. Or mess-to-be. You have an object in the bathroom called a tub. USE IT! And abuse it, too. Once your little one grows old enough to manage his or her own bath, let 'em take one as long as they like. Add generous doses of Popsicles, cocoa, pudding, ripe watermelon, barbecued ribs, whatever, and the goopier the better. So it messes up the bathwater. Who cares? It's easily disposed of when you flick open the drain.

Or keep the tub empty and stage a picnic in there. Again, sloppiness rules. I have found that any authorization a kid can get to legally trash the place, however small that place may be, is beyond a visit to Valhalla. They will be thrilled and overwhelmed, and so busy creating their pre-approved mess that they'll forget about you for the duration of YOUR project.

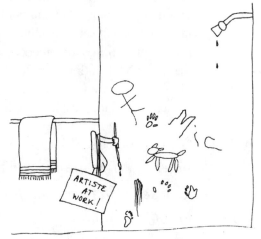

Best yet was a special diversion I gave Mikey when I knew I had some long, drawn-out phone calling to do and Big Sister was off with a class-mate. He wanted to finger-paint, badly. Ordinar-ily, a capital idea. However, it was a cold, wintry day, so sending him outside with a nice, gooey, painty mess you can simply hose down afterwards was not an option that was open to us.

But the bathtub was!

I put him in there, tub empty, with all the finger-paint tubes and jars I could find. A couple of old sponges and paint brushes. And since the bathroom was nice and warm, he had his choice of being clothed or unclothed. My only stipulation was that he wear rubber-soled shoes to keep from slipping. He painted and gooped and slopped the place to his heart's content. He was happy in there for hours, as I discovered when I'd check on him periodically. Aside from occasionally singing something at the top of his lungs, he was relatively quiet. And I got quite a bit accomplished.

This strategy also works well with extended Play-doh adventures. The tub allows a little sculptor to become rather free-wheeling. Just remember not to add tub water or an open drain in the end.

Entertaining The Troops

The only thing you really have to stay on top of in a situation like this is when your little artist needs to get OUT of the tub at the end of the painting session. Believe me, you DO NOT want Young Picasso climbing out, unattended, and coming to find you (tracking half of his or her materials onto the floor or rug en route). If your Artist is old enough, have him or her holler for you to come assist. But that's assuming you'll be within earshot and not behind a closed home-office door. In that case, you take control and set a deadline — say — just 15 minutes more or something. If you think you'll still be too preoccupied concentrating on finishing up, yourself (because that gives YOU a time limit, too), get an egg-timer for your office and let it keep you on schedule. It may not be a reliable strategy simply to keep your eye on your watch.

Remember, too, that the tub makes a great echo chamber . . . if you don't mind the noise, or can sequester yourself far enough away from it for awhile, park them in the empty tub, and let 'em sing and rant and rave. Bring in some little play instruments if you have any, like guitars or keyboards, just as long as you don't include whistles (a little TOO loud), and let them enjoy themselves. Of course, avoid anything with an electrical cord, even if the bathtub is drained. I'd also discourage adding pots and pans or anything else metallic in such a closed space. It turns up the volume too high. You don't want ear damage.

There are ways to get safely reckless in other parts of the house if you need your own time and space to do business. Again, you have to be willing to accept some temporary disruption. And this is certainly NOT the time to be entertaining clients. Take all the cushions off the sofa, or let your child do so, and leave instructions to build something with them. He or she may come up with a house, an obstacle course, a railroad track, or maybe a space ship. (After the Olympics, we had a lot of gymnastic arenas erected in our family room.)

I also keep a few old, ill-fitting and mismatched sheets within easy reach of both my kids. They regularly enlist my help in draping together a tent, or maybe several, in a corner of the living room, behind a couple of big easy chairs. Once I complete construction, they're off and running, and creatively distracted, while I get some work done in my office. At other times, all I'm required to do is point them towards the sheets and they take it from there. Occasionally, I don't even have to do that much, since they'll find all the building materials they need on their own. This approach also works wonderfully on the dining room table. A good-sized sheet will cover the whole works and they can crawl around under it until they drop.

The underlying philosophy here: ANY ideas you come up with that involve changing the place around a little, or better yet, messing it up, will provide an exquisite delight to your child and for a stretch of time, too. It's a kid's version of The Forbidden Fruit.

Another thing to consider, if you want the diversion to be educational and constructive on a different level: You'll probably wind up investing in a second computer for your young 'un. When he or she is very little, there won't be any risk of having your computer monopolized. But when your child grows he or she may be very computer-literate and will fight you for the use of yours — for reading games or drawing programs, and later, for school work. Both of mine are currently addicted to "Sim City" and other town-building programs. Elizabeth's town is "Roses of Barbie." Mikey's is "St. Nick."

Highly-recommended is to set up a special kid's work station or office-ette so yours is left free for you. Provide as many kid-versions of your office supplies as possible. Some of your more kid-friendly ones like envelopes and paper are a good start. You will also automatically nurture all kinds of good study and work habits that way, because your child will come to enjoy doing "MY work while Mommy does hers!"

Letting your children go to pretend-work while you're busy with the real thing, may also keep them from feeling left out while making it easier for you to buckle down. Elizabeth suddenly discovered the wonders of purses. I also lent her my official reporter's microphone to speak into every so often, and old press credentials to wear. Mikey adopted a black derby hat, a pair of Daddy's shoes, and his old, worn-out, emptied appointment book the moment Daddy bought himself a new one. This works magnificently with an old, cast-off attaché case as well. (This is called Advanced Dress-Up 201).

Don't lull yourself into complacency by assuming you'll be able to get a lot done while your little one is napping. Those naps are NEVER long enough for what YOU need to attend to. Often you're going to be too worn out to crank at maximum efficiency and may just "cave in" at those times. You'll probably have to wait until your child is old enough to be at school for a day-long stretch.

Don't lull yourself into complacency by assuming you'll be able to get a lot done while your little one is napping.

You might even find yourself deflating completely while the children are at school, and doing most of your mundane business management WAY after hours, like 24-hour banking and other transactions over the phone or on-line. Even household business like the grocery shopping you could never work in during the day can be done this late, provided there's someone reliable at home to keep watch while you're gone. Or, it may be possible to place an order on-line, if such service is available at a supermarket near you. Will THAT ever save you steps.

The only time you can regularly count on long spans of uninterrupted time to work will be after your little one is asleep for the night. You'll wake up one day to realize that your schedule — that may once have been so predictably nine-to-five — has now gone around the clock and back. Or as I've discovered while pulling yet another near-all-nighter trying to tie up loose ends — every time I turn around, it's three o'clock in the morning.

You may have to consider a part-time helper in the home if you can't organize baby-duty relays with your mate. You'll probably find that your first appointments of the day will be with your husband or baby-sitter, to coordinate who's on active "kid watch" and when. Make a habit of posting schedules on the refrigerator door, the inside of the front door, the outside of your office door, the bathroom mirror, on the phone, or in a phone machine message as to what you'll need, when, and for how long. Here, again, is where that beeper and cellular phone system I described earlier will pay off.

And I did mention baby-sitter. I grit my teeth as I suggest this, because the ideal situation is Mom-home-with-kid. Or Dad-home-with-kid. Or both, if you can swing it. Not a parent substitute. However, realities often dictate that nannies, baby-sitters, and day-care set-ups may have to be examined and tapped into. Hopefully, only temporarily.

Determine how much you'll need and how much you can afford. Do you have enough room for the helping hands to come to you, or do you have to go to them? Every day of the week, or a few days? All day or just part of it? Better yet — do you have relatives (Grandma!) living nearby and able to pitch in? Are you in a neighborhood where a few stay-at-home moms pool their

You may have to consider a part-time helper in the home if you can't organize baby-duty relays with your mate.

resources and you can join in? If not, could you start such an arrangement? Or, do you get REALLY bold and decide that the home business you always dreamed of will be — a day care center? Having a child will impact your evenings profoundly. Including going out to eat.

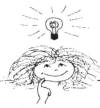

Tips To Remember

✓ There are many approaches to keeping your child occupied and entertained while you do business at home.

✓ Sometimes you can relocate your kid — to Grandma's, a friend's house, or out with Daddy.

✓ Give your child an art project, with lots of crayons, paper, and other supplies.

✓ Your child can play outside without constant supervision — ONLY IF he or she is old enough, it's in a secure BACKyard, and not near a pool, dangerous tools, or on a balcony. And just for a little while at a time.

✓ Many interesting outdoor activities involve making a mess, whether it's with food, mud, finger-painting, chalk, or the garden hose (which the child should not be left alone with unless he or she is older).

✓ Child-pleasing indoor activities can include books, puzzles, selected home videos on TV — the ones starring your kid are best of all.

✓ Any activity that will amuse your child is likely to amuse the neighbor's children, a client's children, or the kids of a fellow frazzled working mom, who could use a breather, herself. The kids are sure to find plenty of distraction in each other's company, which should give YOU a breather, too.

✓ You gain an ally by helping another mom this way. She'll no doubt be someone able to return the favor if you get in a bind.

✓ Some of the most popular indoor activities are those that mess things up. They can also be contained.

✓ Try a "leaf" pile of torn-up grocery bags, a construction project with the sofa cushions, a tent-making project with some old sheets, a finger painting spree in an empty bathtub (make sure the child wears rubber-soled shoes to keep from slipping), or a sing-a-long in there.

✓ When he or she is older, your child will love a LONG bath. In all tub games, you should supervise, but if the kid's older, you don't have to be on constant watch. It helps be within ear-shot, though. And you can set a timer in your office if you think you'll become too absorbed in your work.

✓ Beware the indoor messes you DON'T contain; especially those involving food. You invite ants. Kids are especially adept at these, and can scatter crumbs of all kinds virtually everywhere.

✓ Your child will eventually want or need a computer of his or her own. Dress him or her in some of your clothes and "play office" while you work. Set him or her up with a work station or desk with a few office supplies YOU can spare.

Chapter 12

The Working Mom As A Novelty Act

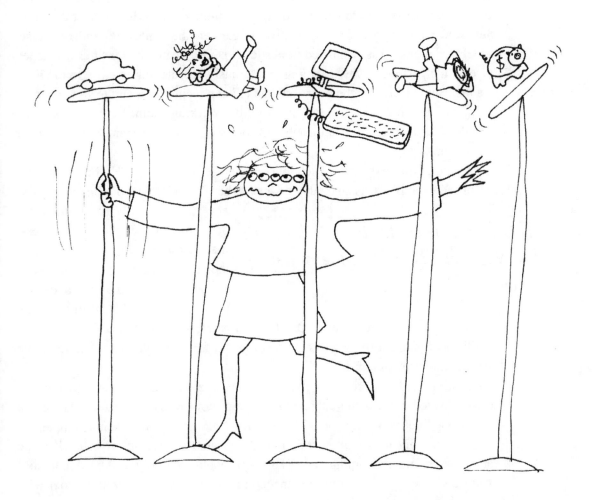

I never realized how one of the regular acts on the old "Ed Sullivan Show" would come to symbolize working motherhood for me.

On the show a man would come out on stage and stand behind a row of tall sticks. Beside him was a table with a stack of plates on it. His mission was to grab a plate, set it on top of one of the sticks and start it spinning there. He'd repeat that until there were spinning plates on top of all of the sticks at the same time. And, of course, the tension mounted as he hurried from stick to stick, because by the time he reached the end, the first plate was wobbling precariously, threatening to crash to the floor in a thousand pieces. So the poor soul had to keep racing back and forth to keep all the plates spinning. That, to me, sums up the working mom. I can still hear the relentless saber dance music throbbing furiously behind our frantic plate-spinner (a.k.a. yours truly).

The end of the first week of school (for not one but now BOTH of my children) is a prime example. It is shakedown week, when I accelerate from just worrying about my schedule to juggling three of them at once. I've tried several maneuvers to get them ready for their day, and me for mine. Do I wake up earlier and do me first, and them afterwards, or do I steal an extra few minutes sleep, then work my preparations in between each of theirs? The various deadlines of your morning will help sort this out for you if you let them. Don't be afraid to experiment a little.

There is a very strong likelihood that you will NEVER get caught up. At least not completely.

I finally made peace with myself about one internal rat race that every self-motivated, high-speed-achieving working mom will have to face. There is a very strong likelihood that you will NEVER get caught up. At least not completely. Unless you want to drive yourself into the ground or reprogram yourself to be satisfied with merely coming close. That's probably the best you'll be able to do. I promise you, even when you've managed to move heaven and earth to your will, you'll find it worked out perfectly for about two or three nanoseconds. Because the minute you get a firm handle on whatever it is, there will arise a whole host of new complications to sort through.

Here, for better or worse, is how to move into at least a suburb of "Perfection-ville," when you see no chance of ever finding its Civic Center:

There are disciplines you follow at work that can be applied at home and will work well. *Working ahead*, for example. In my job at the AP, it was usually always a day's worth, at least for the predictable parts of my duties. So if a breaking story suddenly threw my routine to the dogs, my routine assignments were already researched, written, recorded, produced, in the can, and fed in to the folks in Washington.

One of many times that paid off for me was when I was downtown at the bureau, taking advantage of a slow news day to work maybe TWO days ahead. Everything was "steady as she goes." Mercifully uneventful. Until the outside line rang in the studio. It was Elizabeth's *What can I say? PLANNING is everything.* pre-school, which let out at noon. It was 12:30 and she hadn't been picked up. Seems her dad had an urgent business meeting which was taking longer than expected. He was stuck in there, for a couple of hours, and unable to leave.

I thanked the "slow-news-day angel" as I hurriedly logged off the computer, scooped up my kit bag and the mail I hadn't had time to open all day, grabbed my car keys, and raced for the exit. The slow-news-day angel just happened to be on good terms with the smooth-commuting-angel that day, and even the freeway was benevolent. I made it all the way across town in a record 20 minutes.

What can I say? PLANNING is everything, Especially when working ahead is part of it.

At home, that means exploiting the night before. Lay out the proper kids clothes, assemble the lunch, sign the field trip release form, inspect the backpack for the extras needed the next day; write the check for whatever school expense has to be covered this week. That's when you find out if the proper clothing is ready to go or needs to be washed. Or a button replaced. The night before is where you fix all those

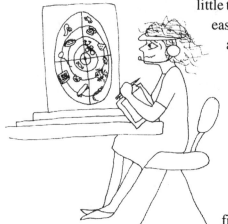

little things. That's also when you bathe the kid, because that can ease them into bedtime, and you don't have to rush as much as you would in the morning. Set the backpack and whatever else gets toted to school the next day right by the front door, with your briefcase or portfolio, so you almost trip over it all when you head out. Chances are you won't go off and forget it!

Use ANY time you have, AHEAD OF TIME, to your advantage. You don't know how grateful you'll be that you did! When packing a lunch, or a snack, don't do just one. Do several at the same time. A half-dozen sandwiches, five of which you can freeze for later. A bunch of celery and/or carrots at once — not just a single serving. Try some of those bulk packages of ready-cut vegetables from which you can grab a handful in a hurry. A handful of grapes in each of several little bags. Other bulk packs of everything from juice boxes to cookies to string cheese will also be MOST useful.

Round up, wash, and pair up ALL the little socks you can find. If you set aside extras of any essential, one of those extras will save you in a last-minute crisis. When my daughter began wearing a uniform, we bought her five blouses; then I hid one. In an emergency, it's there, looking bright and new, for the inevitable day of a visiting dignitary or class photo (when I may have failed all my good intentions the night before).

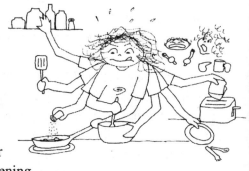

I experienced one of those last-minute crises during shakedown week. The first week of school was also the week leading up to the Emmys — another big news event for me. (You can count on this sort of thing happening during a crucial time for your children.) I was so exhausted that I simply "caved in." Naturally, it was on one exceptionally critical night. Along with all the rest of the uproar, Elizabeth's first loose tooth decided to come out. Of course we all made a huge fuss over it and prepared it for the Tooth Fairy. That far, I managed. And then I hit the wall.

I awoke spontaneously, about half an hour early the next morning. Fancy that! And suddenly my mind was clicking like a pair of castanets. In a fog of my own semi-completed homework for the Emmys, I remembered the things I hadn't done for my first-grader the night before! The new school supplies hadn't been put in the backpack. No lunch or snack was prepared. No clothes were laid out. Nor anything else. So there I was, swooping around the house, grabbing some of the things I HAD prepared in multiples a few days earlier — like mated knee socks and Baggies of carrot strips. This was precisely the kind of morning I'd fixed all those extras for. Whew! Not a bit of that spare time was wasted, and I'd covered all bases. Hadn't I? Well, yeah. I think I did. Aren't I something?

And then — OOOOOOOOHHHHHHHHHHHHHHH!!!!!!!! NOOOOOOO!!

Elizabeth's alarm clock was moments away from going off. She may even be waking up; then a stomach-turning realization hit me. I had it on VERY good authority (from an otherwise reliable source), that the Tooth Fairy hadn't been by yet — if you know what I mean. So, another desperate sweep ensued around the house for what the Tooth Fairy needed. And the Tooth Fairy had to get in and get out before getting "busted."

The Tooth Fairy made it by the hair of her chinny-chin-chin. Leaving me wheezing but thankful that I'd prepared at least a few things in advance. Otherwise, we'd have been out of uniform, hungry, and worse, if the Tooth Fairy had blown it, too. Besides,

I'd have hated to be cutting some last-minute celery sticks in a frenzy and wind up with blood drops on my daughter's uniform and my hand all sliced up for the Emmys. This is what I meant earlier, about little things that add up in a big way.

Sometimes it'll be cyberspace to the rescue, allowing you to cut corners electronically. Like the Wednesday my husband and I were both a day behind in answering our E-mail — right after school had resumed from Christmas break (gee, I wonder what WE were busy with). A nasty bout with the winter cold season had just departed, and hadn't yet decided to come back for one last visit

Sometimes it'll be cyberspace to the rescue, allowing you to cut corners electronically.

(which, of course it did — to me — in another week). The Broadcast Film Critics Association put out an urgent call for write-ups for the program of the awards luncheon in two weeks. Could I take the one about Lauren Bacall? Sure! Could I get it done by close of business tomorrow? The program has to be to the printer by Friday. Hey, no sweat. Consider it done.

Ooooooooooooooooooohhhhhhhhhh, brother!

I love Lauren Bacall. I have for years. And I've thoroughly enjoyed seeing some of her films more than once. But, at that precise instant, my mind went totally blank on the reasons why.

I don't suppose it could have been because we were all jolted back on rigid schedules after totally falling off the discipline wagon over the holidays; or feeling a little shaky after the flu, or sponge bathing ourselves while right in the middle of a couple of extensive shower-door replacement jobs; or reorienting to Mikey's recent karate class upgrade (with a more demanding schedule than we'd been used to); or planning Elizabeth's first slumber party for that rapidly-approaching Saturday. At the same time, Bruce was getting more deeply involved in an extensive arts program at church and was knee-deep in organizational meetings, brainstorming sessions, and conference calls.

Late that night, we had time we could redirect toward surfing the Internet for items that gave me ideas, not to mention some welcome memory fresheners! How on earth had I been able to arrange for THAT? Luck, maybe?

NO!!!

I'd "bought" myself extra time thanks to all that assembly-line sandwich manufacturing and bulk laundry servicing I'd taken care of two nights before when I'd had the chance TO WORK AHEAD!

First thing the next morning, after both kids were delivered to school, I jumped in the car, raced to a bookstore in Hollywood that specialized in theatrical materials, and picked a good Lauren Bacall research tool to supplement further. This was one time when I DID NOT want to rely on my memory if I didn't have to. And I simply HAD to do right by the Grand Dame Bacall. So I welcomed all the back-up I could scrounge. (You will be amazed by how much the cramming you did for exams back in school will pay off later. And you probably thought THOSE particular skills had all but atrophied!)

The 400-word piece got written, accurately, relatively coherently, and with the sentiments I'd developed long before. Just as they were calling to find out where it was, I was putting the finishing touches on it to E-mail it back to them.

ANY shortcut in a storm will help, ESPECIALLY the electronic ones. Because there aren't too many of us who have the time or budget for a messenger service.

Tips 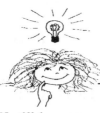 To Remember

✓ You'll become a pro at juggling work, household, and kid activities and needs — mainly because you'll HAVE to.

✓ Scheduling coordination can be honed to a fine art, right from the get-go in the morning. If you have a child to get ready for school, experiment with the timing of breakfast, showering, and dressing by adjusting your own.

✓ Take the pressure off of YOURSELF! Cut yourself slack by realizing you may not get completely caught up.

✓ Many efficiency strategies from work do translate well at home. Especially WORKING AHEAD — preparing for everyone's next-day needs THE NIGHT BEFORE. And in bulk whenever possible. Make or pre-package multiple lunch components ahead of time and then freeze them. Set aside spares of clean clothes for emergencies when you've run out of time to do the laundry.

✓ Investigate the on-line world to help expedite your business and home-management.

✓ Don't assume you can squeeze all of YOUR work in while your kid is napping. That won't ever be enough time and you may need a nap yourself. Longer time spans for work are available while he or she is at school, or asleep for the night.

✓ Make sure you have copies of EVERYBODY'S schedules clearly posted. Including a baby-sitter's or nanny's schedules, too, if you absolutely must have outside help. Everyone's plans and needs should be well-coordinated with everyone else's.

Chapter 13

The Working Mom As A Disappearing Act

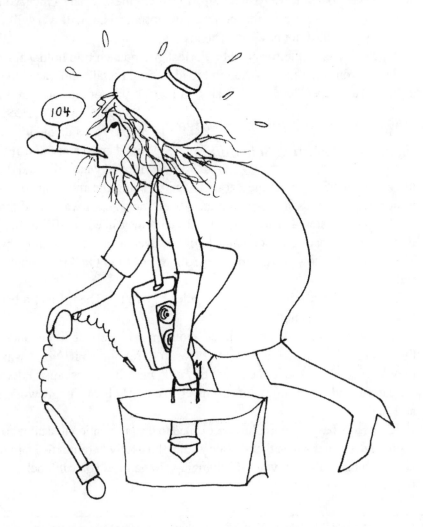

I'm sure you've heard the term "Creative Bookkeeping." Here's a new term you should be prepared to take to heart — "Creative Scheduling." If you've prided yourself at all on being a dedicated professional, the word absenteeism is probably not in your vocabulary. At least up 'til now. Guess what? Once you become a working mom, you and the concept of absenteeism will very likely become well-acquainted, if not new best friends.

I speak, here, as the former Ms. Perfect Attendance title holder for many years running. From the time I started in broadcasting, I totally embraced the philosophy of being "a trouper," one who'd carry on like the post office folks are said to do — through rain, snow, sleet, and dark of

Here's a new term you should be prepared to take to heart — "Creative Scheduling."

night. I was doggedly determined to build my career and my reputation. I loved what I did and didn't want to miss a moment. I Loved the ego-massage of being the morning news companion to hundreds of thousands of commuters every day. And I was afraid that I'd lose it all if I became sick and management decided they liked my fill-in better than me. Besides, broadcasting is one tentacle in the overall octopus of show-biz, is it not? Therefore, that show-biz axiom, "The Show Must Go On," must apply to me, too, right?

For years these were some of my rules to live by. Then, I had a baby. And not too long after that, another one.

Things changed. Like my attitude about my Ms. Perfect Attendance crown, and the realities that made me find good reason to relinquish it. No, it wasn't because they learned about me in the pages of *Penthouse*. It was because I discovered that the careful and judicious use of absenteeism could help me juggle work, home, kids, and sanity.

If you, too, have been mightily dedicated to the proposition that all working women should never miss a day, that — like gliding blissfully barefoot through the house — is something you'll find yourself giving up. Sometimes you can't help it, either.

For one thing, having a kid around means having more germs around. Especially when offspring start school. Then, you have the germs of OTHER offspring around. Everything you've heard about this one is true. Your little one WILL bring home every sniff, sneeze, and sore throat in the classroom, if not the whole school. And if you "luck out" with one kid who remains

Your status as Mom and Chief Cuddler means you are guaranteed to make all their sneezes and wheezes your own.

healthy, your luck will promptly run out if you have a second child. That's what happened with me, once Mikey got here and got rolling. Our hills were alive with the sound of sniffles and we had huge clouds of used Kleenex crowding every wastebasket in the house.

Your status as Mom and Chief Cuddler means you are guaranteed to make all their sneezes and wheezes your own, and in short order, too. It won't make any difference how antiseptically clean your home may be, or how careful you are with your health and vitamin intake. Expect to catch at least some of whatever is going around, whenever it's going around. Or else, I suppose you could always swear off holding them close, smooching them, wiping their noses, or kissing their sweet little "fingies" (yes, the very same ones that were way up their noses a moment earlier). Well, no, I couldn't give up on any of that, either.

Sometimes, a little cold that you'd ordinarily dispense with in a few days will find a way to move in like another member of the family. And it'll move from room to room, too, as it circulates from sibling to sibling to Dad, and most especially, back to you. Trust me, you WILL catch it. Whatever it is. You may be able to avoid some of it, but at least one or two rounds of it WILL find its way to you eventually, no matter how fit you are or how many vitamins you take.

Besides, whatever state of fitness you're in, you will most likely be run down, energy-wise, because as a working mom, you're also in a steady state of being backed up, overloaded, and sleep-deprived. So you're apt to be more susceptible to colds and flu than you ordinarily would be with just yourself or your couplehood to worry about.

I used to dread sick days when I was "on the air" all the time, because, whatever cold or flu came visiting went not towards a sore throat or temperature or runny nose, but severe laryngitis. I could limp through those other miseries, but not when I couldn't talk. You can't function on the radio without a voice, and when mine went south with some traveling bug, the rest of me did, too. Whenever a sore throat would start, I'd find myself hoping it would end there and not spread to the vocal cords. After I had babies, colds of all kinds happened often. Never been sick a day in your life? Just wait until a good dose of parenthood sets in.

Before you go counting up your year's allotment of sick days at the office and start running through it, stop a moment and think ahead. You MUST plan and strategize on this. If you're stuffed up, or crampy, or something, and feel like calling in sick, I strongly recommend you don't if you can stand it at all. Unless you have the kind of job you can take home with you, or you're already telecommuting.

As I mentioned earlier, this applies when you're pregnant, and will be needing to hoard your sick days for the sake of a longer maternity leave. Unless you're stricken with morning sickness that absolutely levels you, or you're so overtired and depleted that the cold you catch is simply unbearable, it's REALLY better to be a trouper now and bank those precious sick days for later.

Besides, you'll never know when you might have an accident like the ones I described awhile back, that marooned me on disability leave for several days. Cases like these may leave you no choice. You're stuck, no matter how ardently you may want to hang in there.

I'll never forget one of the MOST mortifying times when I decided to try to hang on — when the late Jim Henson was in L.A. and available for interview. I loved his work and wanted to make sure I could tell the sprout I was growing inside of me (soon to be Elizabeth) about it as she left her infant stage and learned to love it herself. Since I was pregnant, I didn't want to take any kind of cold medication, and I was determined to stockpile that sick day. I KNEW I could press ahead, and so I did. My sinuses, however, decided not to.

So there we were in the interview room together, midway through our allotted time. I had half my brain on what Jim Henson was saying to me, and the other half focused on where his eyes were. Whenever he'd glance away from me, I'd seize the moment to run a quick finger under my nose to shortstop any runnings. That held me for only so long, though. Soon enough, there came one horrifying moment when I became conscious of an unfamiliar warmth that was oozing down from my nostrils and closing in fast on my upper lip.

OH, MAAAAAAAAAAAAAAANNNNNNNNN!!

I realized I could fake it no longer. I cut my losses and interrupted the interview, begging his pardon and explaining that I simply HAD to excuse myself for a moment and go blow my nose! A sweeter gentleman about this he couldn't have been (probably because HE had kids and undoubtedly plenty of first-hand experience with THEIR second-hand germs). He didn't even look grossed out, bless his heart (DEFINITELY a dad). After the interview was finished, I apologized again, thanked him for being so understanding in the midst of such a disaster, and assured him I wouldn't be shaking hands with him because I didn't want my cold germs to get any closer to him than they already were.

Every time I see "Sesame Street," to this very day, I want to send Jim Henson another mental apology. I don't think I've ever been more humiliated! I think I would have made myself sick over that one if I hadn't been so sick already.

A different twist on that happened to me in the middle of an interview with Connie Stevens. Among other things, she was promoting some benefit work she was doing on behalf of a Native American group. Again, I was pregnant and reluctant to take any medicine, even the over-the-counter types. As she talked, and I rolled tape, I became aware that the sore throat I'd walked in with had started to get creative. Suddenly, there

---

was this excruciating itch in the back of my throat. I tried to clear it by silently swallowing as hard as I could without looking like an idiot or distracting her.

My efforts not only didn't work, but also set off some weird reaction in the middle of my head that immediately started squeezing tears out of my eyes and down my face. Hoping to cover up my total embarrassment, I burbled some lame comment about how I'd been so emotionally moved by what she'd been saying (and her descriptions of her cause WERE quite poignant and heartfelt) that I just couldn't help myself. Sometimes it's enough to make you want to go crawl into a hole somewhere.

Toughing it out, can be an unavoidable trade-off when you're a working mom.

Toughing it out, as you see, can be beyond tough, even though it can be an unavoidable trade-off when you're a working mom. What you need to do is call the doctor (the HEAD doctor for me, sometimes), get a good prescription (make sure it's a SAFE one if you're pregnant) or one of those daytime remedies you can get over the counter (same pregnancy-related precautions apply here, too. DON'T get casual about this) and stagger on in. You DO need to use those sick days, all right, but NOT for you. For your kid.

When your little one has to stay home for a day, it will almost MAKE you sick to leave him or her behind with nanny or baby-sitter (no matter how trusted) or your husband, while you trundle off to the office or a meeting. Regardless of who may be needing you on the job, your kid will need you more, even if just to know you're within "hollering" range, and he or she will want you home. And you'll want to be home. THIS is when you call in sick. Unless, of course, you're willing to make yourself sick with guilt. Suffer through what ails you, but "bail out" for a day if it's for your child. You'll smell like Vicks for awhile, but I promise you that you'll both feel better for it.

And by all means, tailor those phone company commercials (about how technology can be the worker's safest port in a storm) to your own circumstances. Investigate those phone numbers that will ring at your office, home or your cell phone and your beeper, to find you wherever you are. This will allow you to reasonably play hooky and still tend to both job and kid.

He or she will NEED you to be close. Close enough, at times, that you're actually in the bed cuddling while your young 'un suffers. Sometimes, when Elizabeth has had a high fever, and the best answer is a lukewarm bath to cool her down, I tear off my clothes and climb into the tub with her to hold her close. Because she's deliriously upset and needs an emotional cool-down, too. And RIGHT NOW! I learned to keep a spare Mom-sized bathrobe in THEIR bathroom for just such a purpose.

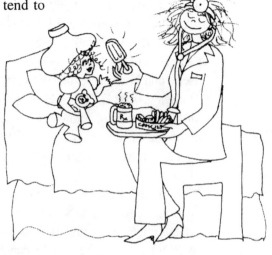

I also learned to keep several stashes of kid medicines and remedies, for fever, sore throat, cough, runny nose, earache, tummy ache, headache, tooth ache (that numbing stuff for teething is ideal), fever blisters, splinters, bruises, bumps, and sprains — in both chewable and liquid form (for sleepytime and needing-to-be-awake time). Plus their favorite magic elixirs — hot cocoa, peppermint tea, and lemon tea. I also highly recommend Popsicles to cool down hot, angry boo-boo's in the mouth, Daddy's ice packs (which have special grown-up cachet for feverish little foreheads), Mom's old T-shirts for a comfort shirt to sleep in, and the King of All Cure-alls: Real Chocolate Marshmallow Pinwheel Cookies. I'm surprised you can still buy THOSE without a prescription.

And if it's at all possible when you have a little patient to care for, try to keep the washing machine empty and ready for action. You may have to clean up a bed-full of sheets and blankets that they got explosively sick upon. These spells always come without warning, and all too often, and they erupt too swiftly to permit a sprint to the bathroom. You'll also have to throw your clothes into that same wash load, no doubt, because they, too, will be a mess. And you won't want, or have time to unload a previous washer-full to accommodate the newest emergency.

Again, I can't emphasize strongly enough the importance of planning your use of sick days. If you're at all concerned about maintaining a professional image to clients or a boss, and still doing right by them, you MUST use these options cautiously and wisely, and NOT TOO OFTEN if you can help it.

I always tried EXTREMELY hard never to call in sick on a Monday or a Friday, unless there was absolutely no way I could avoid it (like those Sunday mishaps I mentioned earlier, that earned me "time-out" in the emergency room). Some people will automatically assume that what you're really up to is a long weekend.

DO NOT exploit sick days, so those to whom you have to report won't be ticked off. And somebody else at the office who's already overworked won't get stuck covering for you AGAIN and, thus, equally ticked off at you. And co-workers WILL start talking. Unfortunately, this does happen. All it takes is one disgruntled colleague who thinks he or she can handle it better, to start a ground swell that's potentially toxic to you.

You HAVE to step gingerly, know your turf, and cover yourself. As I mentioned a few chapters ago, many of the people you work with will be understanding and helpful, especially if they have children and don't have to walk a mile in your moccasins. They've got a few well-worn pairs of their own. But if you're aware of conflicting ambitions around you, think carefully about how liberally you take advantage of these conveniences.

Then, again, if you do it smoothly enough, you'll be setting an example of how juggling can succeed for your co-workers, as well as for yourself. Remember, some young woman coming up behind you may not necessarily be a threat. She could ALSO be wondering if she, too, could handle motherhood AND her profession.

Tips 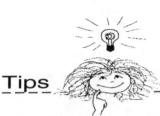 To Remember

✓ Once you become a working mom, you'll likely be needing a few more sick days.

✓ A child in your life means more germs in your life. He or she will bring colds home from classmates — in pre-school and beyond. A SECOND child in your life means a double shot of that, at least. And once germs gain a foothold, they're apt to rage through the whole house and everybody in it.

✓ Expect to be more susceptible, because your general day-to-day condition includes exhaustion, sleep deprivation, and extra stress. Besides, you're the one who hovers closest to the little one, whether he or she is sick or well.

✓ Try not to run through your ration of sick days, even if morning-sickness is hitting you hard, because you're liable to need them MORE — later.

✓ You MUST use your sick days WITH CARE AND DISCRETION. Don't overdo it. Especially if the only sick one is you. If you can soldier on at the office, and save the sick day for later, by all means, do so.

✓ You may prefer to use YOUR sick days to stay home with a sick child.

✓ Make sure you have a full supply of cold and flu medicine, children's Tylenol, and other remedies for little aches and pains.

✓ You'll also need a full supply of excellent fruit and mint teas, sweets for the little sweetheart, and Popsicles for sore little mouths.

✓ Other good "Dr. Mom" prescriptions include Dad's ice packs, Mom's T-shirts, and lots of your own close contact.

✓ Also, make sure your washing machine is ready for use — because you're liable to have to clean up after an explosively sick child.

The Working Mom As A Disappearing Act

✓   Again, be careful and judicious in your creative use of sick days.

✓   DO NOT ABUSE this privilege! Avoid calling in sick on Mondays or Fridays, especially because people will assume you're playing hooky for a long weekend. Remember, your absence will very likely cause a work overload for the folks at the office — and potential hard feelings against you.

Chapter 14

Emotional Rescue

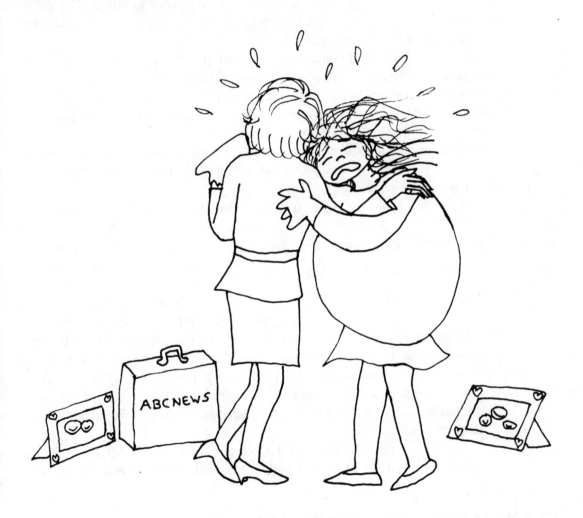

Before I had children, I spent most of my career hoping, striving, and straining to be another Barbara Walters. ANY woman worth her salt in broadcast journalism wants the same thing, even if she's never heard of Barbara Walters. My goal was always in the back of my mind, from the day I signed on at my college radio station and turned the 10-watt transmitter on in the morning to start my first show, until the day I signed off active mode at the AP.

Little did I know that I would reach my goal in sort of a "backdoor" way. And what finally brought me there was *motherhood* and realizing that I'd be willing to give up my career for the sake of more time with my babies. This hit me when I finagled a brief one-on-one with Barbara Walters, after she'd held a press conference to promote another major milestone in her career.

By that time it had become something of a habit of mine to pitch one or two mom-related questions to whatever female celebrity I knew was a mom. Sometimes the answers were revealing personal gems.

I figured that if anyone could, Barbara Walters would know how to handle the working mom's "guilt," *so*, after the news conference ended, I asked her. Her answer was no surprise to me. In fact, I could just as easily have answered for her. First, she heaved a

> *Little did I know that I would reach my goal in sort of a "backdoor" way. And what finally brought me there was motherhood.*

sigh. Then, she smiled in a resigned sort of way, and told me flat out that you never really do handle it — either completely or effectively, while balancing what you need for your own creative sustenance with what your child needs. All you can hope for is to do the best you can. And interestingly enough, she added that the ups and downs of working motherhood were subjects she'd often asked some of the celebrity moms SHE interviewed.

I knew in that instant that I, too, had hit a career milestone. I did MUCH more than just relate. I realized that, in a way, I really HAD become Barbara Walters, after all.

If you are a working mom you will always have that monkey on your back. And you'll have a little catch in your throat when you head out to work leaving your young one behind. You'll be leaving a big part of you behind, too, as you step through the door and wishing you could stay.

And it will follow you around at work, just as your child does at home. As I mentioned awhile back, you WILL wear your heart on your sleeve, right up front with the pabulum or the little nose wipe. And it will gnaw at you at any time.

I took comfort wherever I could. One time I found myself nearly losing it toward the end of an interview with Jaclyn Smith about one of her TV movies. Yes, we had gotten around to Subject A.

Jaclyn has her own version of Elizabeth and Mikey. And we found ourselves trading emotional memories about treasured little gifts, homemade by treasured little hands. Times when they'd go away for the weekend or the night, and it would be the kids acting like the grown ups, being worried about the "basket case" of a Mom they'd left behind. And the children's sto-

You'll have a little catch in your throat when you head out to work leaving your young one behind.

ries that each of us had problems getting through without choking right up. For her it was a little number titled, "I Love You Always," while mine was, "The Velveteen Rabbit."

Ann Jillian was another celebrity who'd become a little mushy at the very mention of her little boy — the child she and her husband had almost given up hope of ever having. She proudly imitated his first attempts at speech, and cooed when I divulged some of my favorite nicknames for my kids. She had plenty of her own for her son. It would have been embarrassing, if we weren't both moms.

Every obit I worked on was a major pull on the heartstrings. And after I became a mom, before it was time to cover a beloved fallen star, whether it was George Burns, Gene Kelly, Raymond Burr, Sammy Davis Junior, Lucille Ball, or Michael Landon, I would want to grab my purse and car keys and run home to hug my little people. To say you're torn can't even begin to describe it. And the extra energy you'll have to find within yourself to stay focused on what pays the bills will tax you, emotionally, even more.

It's difficult to be a working mom. Really hard on the heart. It could be your heart tugging at you when your husband calls, as mine frequently did, with one or the other of our kids getting on the phone saying, "Mommy, are you coming home soon?"

AAAAAAAAAA!!

It could be a thoughtless or unwitting remark from a co-worker about the presence of a baby picture in a communal work area. One such instance left me wondering which one of my kids was Flotsam and which was Jetsam, (as I recall it being worded).

Or it could be the moment when you realize that little person who's pre-empted your emotions can emote right back atcha! It still tears me up a little to recall the first time I realized that Elizabeth started actively and openly loving me back — and during a MOST UN-loving time.

The Gulf War had just broken out. It was only a few days old. And at the ol' AP, everybody's work schedules and assignments were thrown up into the air and right

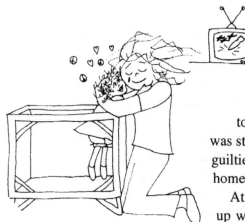

out the window. My closest co-worker in the L.A. bureau was ripped away from his new wife, HER kid, and his daily regional audio duties, and sent cross-country to the Pentagon, and shortly thereafter, on to Saudi Arabia. I was reassigned to hold down the fort for HIM (and all our regional audio affiliates), and had to cut my Hollywood beat by about half. Even so, I was still coming home hours later, every day, and feeling guiltier and guiltier about the longer time I was away from home and high chair.

At home we watched the war on TV so I could keep up with it on a just-in-case mode. I not only wore my beeper, I slept with it on. During weekends, we coped with new and unfamiliar feelings of insecurity by moving Elizabeth's playpen into our bedroom so she'd be close by when she was awake.

I'd spend hours leaning against the corner of that playpen so I could be face-to-face with her whenever she felt like standing up. And as I watched the tense overseas drama of Schwarzkopf versus Saddam, I began a bigtime romance at home with a little girl. I'd spend many emotional moments worrying about friends covering the battlefields, and what the whole affair meant to planetary peace, and even MORE emotional moments basking in the affections of my daughter. She'd prop herself up in her corner of the playpen, where she'd reach out to hug my neck, stroke my cheeks, and smile at me with a look of the sweetest, most comforting empathy I've ever seen. If the big one had dropped right then, I'd have had everything I needed.

I'll never get over the guilt I felt after the first REALLY long day I'd spent at work after I made the move to Planet Baby. It was the first Oscar nomination day following Elizabeth's birth. Not only was it within the first month after maternity leave, it was also the longest stretch of hours I had ever spent

I'll never get over the guilt I felt after the first REALLY long day I'd spent at work after I made the move to Planet Baby.

away from her in any one day's time. To make matters worse, it was Valentine's Day. So, with broken-hearted visions of my little Valentine having spent the day in someone else's arms, I stopped by a gift shop on the way home and picked up a teddy bear for her. It still gets me, right in the stomach, that THIS particular teddy bear (of all the teddy bears she already owned) became Fraula, her instant favorite. And that — years later — we still celebrate Valentine's Day as Fraula's birthday.

It's also difficult on the resolve to be a working mom. For many reasons. Not just keeping your eyes on your work when you're on the job, but keeping it together while off-duty, making sure you're doing as good a job with the little one. As I said before, there's no formula for motherhood as there are with many jobs and work procedures.

Trying to maintain my own "boss-ship" at home is some of the toughest work I've ever attempted. Sometimes Elizabeth generates the "grief," and at other times it's her little brother. And at times it's both of them in collusion. I'll try any approach that works, and they all work at one time or another. Requesting. Demanding. Nagging. Screeching. Retiring to my bedroom and closing the door, declaring before I leave that, "I'm just NOT going to stay around here and be part of this while you're not minding." Or closing myself into my office — not to work but to HIDE. Or count to ten, as it were.

Or using "the position," a behavior modification technique recommended to me by a psychologist friend in cases where the child is determined to remake *The Exorcist* for you, complete with a head you expect to see turning completely around, and pea soup pouring from the mouth. Elizabeth never needed this, but Mikey did.

What you do is sit down on the floor, cross-legged, with him seated too, encaged in your legs. If necessary, you can sit with your back up against the wall (an appropriate match for your feelings in those circumstances) so that his thrashings won't throw you off balance. And around the upper half of him you wrap your arms, so that he's not so much restrained as contained. Nothing tight. He can move and breathe very easily but he can't flail, hit, kick, lurch, OR most importantly, escape.

And there he has to stay until he mellows out and returns to the human race again. He can yell and scream in outrage and protest as loudly as he wants. You, meanwhile, have your face close behind his head, where you're in position to be able to speak quietly in his steaming little ear, urging him to cool it. It does work quite well to gain control of a bullheaded wee one.

Sometimes I try to "clever" them out of it. I shamelessly invoke Santa Claus, or their hard-earned treasure tickets that are now seriously at risk. Or the already-scheduled play date or sleep-over they're about to sacrifice to the misbehavior angel. When I bark out directives that may not be meeting with satisfactory compliance, sometimes I follow it with "... and THAT'S an order!" This usually brings a favorable response.

Other times, I state flatly that "you HAVE to do my bidding. I AM the queen. I outrank you. You are only the princess (or the prince, depending on who is being the royal pain at the moment)." I particularly enjoy moments when they're being extra demanding, or uncooperative but not to the point where I'm getting severely annoyed. Then, I calmly repeat MY demands, and admonish them that they WILL respond with a "yes, oh Mother, my Queen." And, guess what? That's exactly what they do.

Unless, of course, I get fired. Mikey has fired me several dozen times by now, telling me I'm NOT his mother anymore, or that he will never love me again. Until a few minutes later and maybe a cookie or something gets in there, too. Or he decides he would LIKE one. Or, he's otherwise distracted. Then I'm rehired.

Or better yet, he gives me a big, juicy, angry raspberry. Usually with lots of spit-spray. Nowadays, I try to keep my wits about me enough to get a Polaroid of it, or even better, a video. As angry as we both may be at that moment, it only takes one good look at the resulting photo to snap me right out of it. Those pictures never fail to start me laughing.

Tom Snyder told me once that he could really relate. By now, it was to his grand-daughter. He described the first time she'd spent about eight hours visiting his home. He was baby-sitting so her parents could have a day off. She was about two-and-a-half at the time. And he adored her. He always counted the minutes until they were together. But this eight-hour stay of hers was proving to be, well, just a little bit too much for Grandpa. He called a close pal who also has grandchildren and sought advice, wondering if it was normal to want to start counting the minutes 'til she LEFT!

By the way, the friend, he reported, answered absolutely yes. Yeah. I know how it is.

Every now and then, those conflicting feelings arise within me, toward both of my little people, my son in particular. Many times, while "insisting" him into bed for the 59th time that night, I will turn to him and say with exasperation, "WHAT am I gonna do with you, eh?" And Mikey will chirp right back "you're gonna love me!"

Tips To Remember

✓ Once you become a working mom, you will be beset with divided loyalties — pitting your dedication to your work against your devotion to your child. The emotions of this conflict will tear at you constantly. And you'll have a conflicting image — the focused professional versus the mush-pot mom.

✓ Be prepared to fight the emotions generated by the plaintive call from home, with Little One asking when you're coming home. Not all your co-workers can be expected to understand or sympathize with this, so you'll be coping with it on your own.

✓ You'll also have plenty of conflicting feelings toward your child — depending on the changeable nature of his or her obedience.

✓ You'll develop your own versions of what works to bend him or her to your will, ranging from outshouting the kid to banishment to the bedroom, matching wits, muscles, and patience (see the discussion of "The Position") — in effective containment of an angry or contrary child.

✓ Be prepared for your kid's attempts to outsmart you, "cute" you into giving in, or play you off against your spouse. It's essential that you and their dad coordinate your responses and resolve so one of you doesn't inadvertently countermand the other.

✓ If the behavior goes berserk, get revenge: snap a Polaroid of the insolent face or raspberry that your child has punished you with, or videotape a tantrum. The humiliation factor for your child and the amusement factor for you should lighten the mood considerably.

Chapter 15

What On Earth Do You Mean "Time For You"?

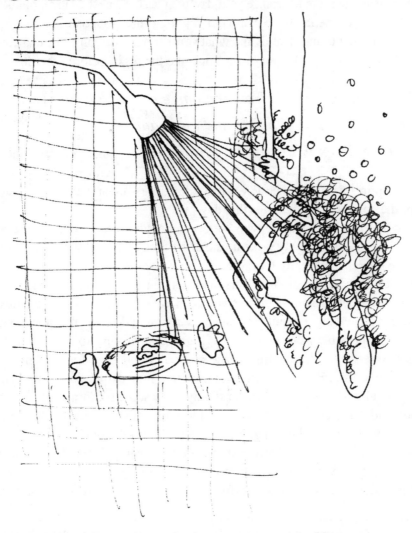

I noted earlier how important it is to nail down what time in the morning you can use for yourself. I've come to appreciate the shower more than ever before. I heartily recommend it for thinking time. If you do it early enough, nobody else is awake and needy yet. You have breathing room to arrange your day, or at least the next 30 to 60 minutes.

Make your mental lists, plan your driving route, your sales pitch, your schedule of appointments and errands and what you'll wear. You can coordinate them all with the business you took care of for your tike the night before. An ideal opportunity occurs during those conditioner treatments that you're supposed to leave on for a few minutes before rinsing off. Instead of just standing there with goop on your head, work your brain. Or go the other way and use that time to clear your mind, to steel yourself for the commotion ahead for that day.

> *I've found that driving to and from the office or assignment can offer a little peace and quiet and time for thinking. Even while fighting traffic.*

While I'm one of those who prefers to do advance work the night before, other working moms routinely wake up a half-hour early to deal with it. Still others like to wake up REALLY early for morning runs or workouts. On rare occasions, I do, too, but you have to be a morning person by nature to do this on a regular basis, and I am not. Nevertheless, some working women swear by this strategy. And I must admit that there is something tranquilizing about the morning dew and the quiet house.

As impossible as it seems, I've found that driving to and from the office or assignment can offer a little peace and quiet and time for thinking. Even while fighting traffic. Because, with apologies to all the carpooling campaigns out there, you're alone in the car with your thoughts, or some soothing music to mellow you out, and that can be very beneficial. Or work off some steam with heavy metal or oldies with familiar lyrics against which you can belt your brains out. Or a talk radio station with some blowhard host at whom you can yell and hurl insults.

ANY time you can beg, borrow, or steal for yourself, either to get some extra things done, catch your breath for a moment, or exercise stress demons, will end up helping you and everyone you live and work with. Some kinds of carpools can actually enhance this, too. My kid's school carpool gave me an extra hour or so, every other week, as long as it lasted.

You can also make your lunch hour start working for you in self-indulgent ways that improve your mental health. The longer a lunch break you have, the more time you have to go shopping, read, take a leisurely stroll, or even stretch out for a little while and do nothing. Some women with an hour break in the middle of the day decide to exercise rather than eat. They find a place to work out near the office and take advantage of it. Still others get a few like-minded colleagues together and set up their own exercise classes for that hour. Or they designate it as mere playtime and gossip over lunch with some friends. Then again, if you feel motivated to do something constructive, go with the urge to run a couple of your less-complicated errands now, like stopping by the cleaners or gassing up your car. You may not have a chance to do them later, when you thought there'd be time for it.

You can also make your lunch hour start working for you in self-indulgent ways that improve your mental health.

Do not, however, assume that an activity as ambitious as a haircut, or visit to the chiropractor or acupuncturist can also qualify as a therapeutic lunchtime out. Nails, maybe. But I've found you can't always count on your carefully-scheduled appointment to start on time, and the day you have no margin for error is precisely the day something is bound to go wrong.

Your lunch hour is also not the best time to book a massage or a facial, because you'll be too pulverized to focus on work when you get back to the office, and all that pore-cleansing will leave you red and puffy-looking. Lunch breaks that you want to use for other reasons MUST allow you a reliable return time. Far better to postpone those until a day when you can leave work early and squeeze them in on your way home.

Or investigate manipulative scheduling. Find out if it's possible to adjust your hours a little. Flex-time may compound its value because it will allow

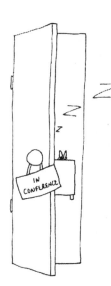

you to avoid the conventional commuter hours, so your trip to and from the office won't take as long. You can use that extra time for other things. Another option worth exploring, provided it's not forbidden by union regulations or something, is whether you can work straight through your day and take your lunch at the end. Which really means you get to leave an hour earlier.

You may soon find yourself boiling down all your lists of stuff-to-cram-into-any-spare-moment into only one simple activity. Catnapping. Whenever possible. Because the standard good night sleep will become something like a driver's license: a privilege, not a right.

By the time I became a mom, I realized that my 13-or-so years of working in news beforehand had been an ideal boot camp for the rigors of motherhood. I was almost always assigned the morning drive shift, which starts on the air no later than 6:00 a.m. You have to be present and accounted for in the newsroom a lot earlier to prepare. I eventually grew accustomed to sleep deprivation — a natural state of affairs for parenthood, too. There are all those round-the-clock feedings and fussy spells when the baby's brand new.

When you're back at work you've added your job, in effect, as another kind of baby in need of your attention. So, you'll be worrying about everything that can possibly be worried about, which — you guessed it — keeps you up at night.

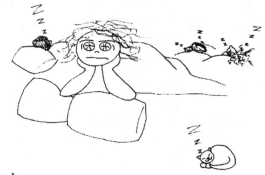

Expect at least a few blowups with your mate that really won't reach hurricane strength until at least 2:30 a.m. You'll be dangling off each other's frayed ends because that lack of sleep is going to take its toll on your man also. And as your little one gets older and more mobile, he or she is liable to pay you visits in the middle of the night for many reasons. Needing a change of diaper or sheets, or mumbling "my feet are cold," "I can't find my Teddy bear," "I wanna cuddle," or "there's a monster in my room."

You'll be faced with episodes like this on both ends of your "night's sleep" and in the middle of it. Think it'll all die down by morning? Not on your life! Often I've been awakened WAY before I want to be. On rare occasion, one of my precious visitors will wet OUR bed. MY side of OUR bed, of course.

Most often, I find myself being crowded to death. One of them is on either side of me, each pressing towards the other. Those take-no-prisoners elbows are drilling them-selves into my sides. My mouth and nostrils are suddenly full of locks of hair. Or feet, if they've changed directions, as they frequently do. Legs are flung wildly all over my body. And the kids' presence means their favorite sleeping companions (Elizabeth's white teddy bear, Fraula, and Mikey's black velveteen kitty cat, whose name is Sprout Brussel Housekeep Initial — Sprout for short) have forced their way in, too. For me, no comfortable position is even remotely attainable. And if I move too much, I risk waking one or both of them, and then my peace and quiet, however pulverized, is completely "outta here."

All of that and more will rank your pursuit of sleep right up there with the Quest for the Holy Grail. It may well be years before you can anticipate a full eight hours sleep, at which time you may be out of the habit of sleeping that long a stretch without interruption.

- -

What On Earth Do You Mean "Time For You"?

My hat remains off to some of the actress-moms I came across, who muscled through, or back to, horrendously-demanding gigs while trying to stay on the Mommy track. And how they, too, battled exhaustion, as resolutely as any of the rest of us do.

Kate Mulgrew told me of being barely able to drag herself home after wrapping one season finale on "Star Trek: Voyager" — with its 14-to 16-hour days. She said she trudged in through the front door, home to her young sons, and just laid down flat — right on the floor.

Bette Midler had the fortitude to make sure her own show went on (probably through sheer force of will) in a demanding promotion tour for her film *Big Business*. But as she sat with us in the interview, I wasn't the only one who noted how depleted she seemed to be. We soon learned that she'd just recently recovered from the physical and emotional upheaval of a miscarriage.

And Jane Seymour. Now THERE's the closest thing to Superwoman I've ever seen! The last time I interviewed her, she was gracious enough to squeeze me in for an interview, on location WAAAAAAYYY out in the sticks, miles from any soundstage, while filming "Dr. Quinn, Medicine Woman." She was playing a serious "Beat the Clock" game of her own. She and the rest of the cast and crew were rushing to complete as many episodes as they could while Dr. Mike still had a waistline. Because Seymour herself had just discovered she was pregnant with twins, and was trying to hold up against a case of double-barreled exhaustion. In heavy costume, in the heat of summer, trying to get well into the next season while most other shows were still on hiatus from the last one.

And she could still stand up. Even though a chair in the shade was always kept open for her. And here she was, concerned about whether I was comfortable and insisting that a chair be found for me, too. And all I had to drag around with me was a big purse and my recording equipment.

Things like that always made me wonder what on earth I was complaining about. Oh, yes, I forgot. Working mom's exhaustion. Guess I was just too worn out to remember clearly . . .

You'll find that catnaps will help you make do. WHENEVER you can find an excuse to work them in, TAKE ONE! And you can make some of them do double duty. If you can only finagle 15 or 20 minutes, you can compound the pleasure with some aromatherapy. I've discovered a delightful little eye-mask filled with scented herbs that seems to amplify the relaxation. It's small enough to take to work if you think you can put your feet up during lunch. If you anticipate you'll doze too deeply for too long, just keep a travel alarm clock in one of your desk drawers. At home, a fragrant candle can also enhance that precious time-out. This one's best if you're alone, though, because small flames and small fingers do NOT mix.

You'll find that catnaps will help you make do. WHENEVER you can find an excuse to work them in, TAKE ONE!

It IS conceivable, though, that somewhat longer escapes, and realistic ones, too, can and will come your way as your little sprout grows. If you can JUST HOLD ON 'til then. And boy, can you use them to get things done. Work or otherwise.

You might use some of that time to shore up the bonding with your man — that's most certainly been left begging since you had a baby. Because that baby moves right up to the head of the class on your list of personal VIPs as soon as he or she arrives.

Once Elizabeth and Mikey were both old enough that we could, in good conscience, leave them behind, for short spurts, in the care of Grandma or the nanny we had for awhile, we'd do so. For a brief stretch, we even made a routine of it on Saturday mornings, where we'd go out on our rounds (errands of every imaginable kind) and then to lunch. We were alone where we could sit, and talk about adult things, completely uninterrupted. No napkins or spoons to pick up. No multiple excursions to the bathroom to chaperone. No furtive need to flag down a waiter for some emergency drink-spill mop up. It was my little weekly oasis from work and kids for a few mellow hours. Yeah, right.

BEEP-BEEP-BEEP-BEEP-BEEP-BEEP-BEEP-BEEP-BEEP-BEEP-BEEP!

It was the bureau downtown. I responded on our cell phone. It was the bureau CHIEF. Oh-oh. Whatever it was, I didn't do it! Actually, he was in the office pitching in as the on-duty folks tried to get to the bottom of the latest breaking typhoon in the ongoing Michael Jackson case. We had to get in touch with Jackson's attorney, Howard Weitzman, right away, the chief said. Weitzman wasn't returning anybody's calls from the bureau that morning, and the developing story was urgent. He said he knew I'd had enough conversations with Weitzman in my own pursuit of the story that Weitzman would probably recognize my name and call me back. So would I try as soon as it was feasible, even though it was a Saturday?

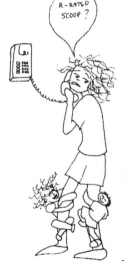

As soon as we got home, I called Weitzman's number, identified myself, and he DID indeed take my call, which I DID indeed appreciate. However, he didn't want to talk too much on the latest prickly development. He told me that because he liked me and thought I had dealt with him fairly, he wasn't going to hang up on me. But at that moment, he was in a hurry to take HIS kids out somewhere, and didn't have much else to say about anything, much less our story.

Well, at least, I got a rather wordy version of "no comment" out of him, which was better than nothing at all. I let Weitzman go tend to his kids (sorry, I couldn't relate ONE BIT to that, could I?), as mine were both subdividing me, each trying to climb up one of my legs, while I was on the phone with Weitzman. If he'd known what was really going on, on my end of the line, I'll bet Howard Weitzman would have appreciated the comic relief.

In one way I'm actually glad that he wasn't willing to give me too much information. It's rather "dicey" to be asking questions about an alleged child molestation case when you've got two "itty bitties" hanging on you, and thus well within earshot. Besides, if Weitzman had agreed to elaborate, I would have asked him to do it on tape. So I'd have rushed for my tape recorder and clip leads so I could record his comments for the record — and probably would have fallen all over my kids in the process.

So much for trying to get reacquainted with your mate — while your clothes are still on.

Or, heyyyyy, there IS that OTHER valiant attempt (or near miss, around our house). You and your mate CAN get reacquainted . . .

PHYSICALLY!

THESE moments do indeed get more and more rare as you sink deeper into parenthood. I guarantee you all those dog-eared jokes and clichés about Child-Walking-In-On-Mom-And-Dad-Having-A-Bit-Too-Much-Fun aren't fiction or exaggeration. They're FULLY fact-based. Without going into details, I can personally testify that this is so.

Then again, you may spend those time-outs on sleep, pure and simple. For example, as he or she gets older, your child will start discovering the joys of sleep-overs. A grandparent's house, or that of a favorite aunt and uncle and/or cousins are good places to start, before you work up to one at a friend's house. If you have one child, one sleepover is your ticket to a night off. And in our case, Grandma agreed to go double or nothing from time to time, and have them both over at once.

Bruce and I, thinking ahead, carefully coordinated one of these on a night when we each had separate business activities in the evening. After those were wrapped up, we reasoned, we'd use that time on a joint work project, and write and edit the night away with abandon. We salivated over the prospect of no interruptions or midnight wanderings. No aggressive lobbying campaigns to postpone bedtime 'til later and later. We could work as long as the inspiration lasted, without worrying about morning obligations. Since it was during everyone's summer vacation, we could count on sleeping in.

And at ANY point during that time, we could . . . Well . . . YOU know . . . What any self-respecting and emotionally-attached male and female might do if given a few moments alone together without intrusions! Hey, you do what you can.

We both reconnoitered after the early evening's events. The entire rest of the night stretched out before us as languorously as an old-time silver screen siren. Like it was with Burgess Meredith in that classic "Twilight Zone" episode, temporarily blessed with all the time he wanted after the rest of the world that so annoyed him was lost to a nuclear bomb.

Guess what we wound up doing with all that luxurious free time? Yep, sleeping. We made burgers in the kitchen while it was still relatively early, and then we just crashed flat out. Pathetic, but true.

I'm always looking for good meltdown insurance in cases where the little darlings have gotten to me so badly I start to think I'm overdosing on them. Or I'm just so sleep-starved that I'm emotionally suffocating toward everybody. Sometimes it's as simple as remembering the "dirt nap" reference Jonathan Winters once made while telling me about the satisfaction of life and family that he will finally take to his grave. That description always lightens me up. Might as well not complain, since I'll be facing my own "dirt nap" soon enough.

This is the time to excuse yourself, and spend 10 or 15 minutes with one of those disgusting-but-refreshing at-home facials. The absurdity value of this is an unexpected dividend all by itself. These masks make you look so temporarily ridiculous that they'll make you laugh — which you may need more desperately than any skin treatment.

Keep your eyes peeled and your mind open and you'll be able to shave off little chunks of time all over the place — for many valuable uses. But you'll have to analyze some of these possibilities carefully. What may seem like a great shortcut at first may turn out not to be. For example, following the first O.J. trial suggested to me the REAL reason Marcia Clark may have changed her hair.

At first she probably figured that a permanent would save her time fussing with her hair in the morning. It may indeed have done this for awhile. But she's a working mom, too, and she probably discovered — as I did myself when I had a similar one — that a permanent can also be a hassle. It has to be maintained, which means you're a slave to a long salon appointment on a regular basis. Too often, you may not have that big a chunk of time to set aside for this. And, it may not be practical to take all your paperwork and cell phone with you to the hairdresser's. And these things, if done properly, cost money Marcia may have preferred to use for a kid's birthday, assuming she hadn't already spent it on fines from Judge Ito.

I saw a bumper sticker recently that sticks just as well to my situation — something to the effect of "a mother is a working woman." Add motherhood to the job equation you already have, and you will REALLY be a working woman. On double overtime. Your pay will be in kisses, lots of laundry, and a whole new appreciation of your whole new set of skills. It will leave you exhausted, often frustrated, yet deeply satisfied at the same time. And there will be moments when you'll juggle so much so effectively, and avert so many crises, that you may become convinced that you really are a Superwoman. Mind you, you aren't. But at the same time don't forget that guy on "The Ed Sullivan Show" and his spinning plates. He rarely broke any.

Tips 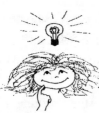 To Remember

✓ Believe it or not, you CAN find some precious time just for yourself if you know where to look, regardless of the stress you're under as a working mom.

✓ Your morning shower (before everybody else gets up and starts making demands of you) is a good time to plot out your day, your responsibilities, and your schedules. Or you can simply use that time alone to clear your head.

✓ You can fit in all sorts of private pleasures or unfinished business if you're willing to get up early enough. That includes a morning run or workout.

✓ While carpooling can offer you some intermittent spare time, commuting alone in your car can provide some good therapy (via singing to or shouting at the radio).

✓ Lunch breaks offer time to run simple errands, pursue a change of pace, or even a nap. Make sure your desk has a small alarm clock to keep you from oversleeping. DO NOT try to squeeze in more extensive appointments — with the doctor or facialist. These errands can't be counted on to start OR end on time.

✓ Investigate creative scheduling, such as flex-time, and/or a movable lunch period that you may be able to take at the end of your day (thus making it shorter).

✓ The search for some personal time will extend to the search for some decent shut-eye. Or for rest, in any event, from the extra burdens, demands, and stresses of your dueling obligations — your job and your child. Catnaps will become increasingly important during the day, since a full night's sleep may not be an available option. Be prepared to be awakened, maybe more than once, by your child, needing you for a variety of reasons.

✓ The same sleep deprivation will also afflict your man — and you know what THAT means . . .

✓ Fortify your catnaps with aromatherapy to enhance the restfulness and avoid oversleeping by setting an alarm.

✓ Take heart: as your child grows older, you'll have more time. He or she will be in school longer, and will be eligible for sleepovers at a friend's or Grandma's. You might want to use some of the time to get reacquainted with your mate.

✓ It IS true that the intimate part of your relationship can go wanting while you're both so intensely focused on the kid. Said kid is liable to break up a few close encounters of yours unless it's during school or you can lock yourselves in.

✓ Keep your eyes open for mood-raisers that will give you an emotional respite: Find those silly Polaroids of your kid working up a lather. Just about any kid pictures will do. Wear one of those boldly-colored mudpack facials around and have a giggle. And why not — keep collecting those short-cuts. Frazzle-busters come in all shapes and sizes, and are apt to pop up anywhere, and at any moment.

✓ Remember above all else: WHEN ALL IS SAID AND DONE, YOU MAY BE FRAZZLED, BUT YOU'RE STILL GOING TO BE OKAY.

Books by Starburst Publishers
(Partial listing—full list available on request)

The Frazzled Working Woman's Practical Guide to Motherhood　　　—Mary Lyon

It's Emma Bombeck meets Martha Stewart meets cartoonist Cathy Guisewite. The author's extensive original cartoon illustrations further enliven a sparklingly humorous narrative, making her a new James Thurber! *Frazzled* is an essential companion for any working woman who thinks she wants a baby, or is currently expecting one. Especially if she could use a good laugh to lighten her load and her worries. This book also offers an innovative update on effective working-mom strategies to women who are already off and running on the "Mommy Track."

(trade paper)　ISBN 0914984756　**$14.95**

God's Abundance　　　—Edited by Kathy Collard Miller

Subtitled: *365 Days to a Simpler Life*. This day-by-day inspirational is a collection of thoughts by leading Christian writers such as, Patsy Clairmont, Jill Briscoe, Liz Curtis Higgs, and Naomi Rhode. *God's Abundance* is based on God's Word for a simpler, yet more abundant life. Similar in style to the best-seller, *Simple Abundance*, but with a Biblical basis. Most people think more about the future while the present passes through their hands. Learn to make all aspects of your life—personal, business, financial, relationships, even housework can be a "spiritual abundance of simplicity."

(hardcover)　ISBN 0914984977　**$19.95**

Revelation—God's Word for the Biblically-Inept　　　—Daymond Duck

Revelation—God's Word for the Biblically-Inept is the first in a new series designed to make understanding and learning the Bible as easy and fun as learning your ABC's. Reading the Bible is one thing, understanding it is another! This book breaks down the barrier of difficulty and helps take the Bible off the pedestal and into your hands.

(trade paper)　ISBN 0914984985　**$16.95**

The Miracle of the Sacred Scroll　　　—Johan Christian

In this poignant book, Johan Christian masterfully weaves historical and Biblical reality together with a touching fictional story to bring to life this marvelous work—a story that takes its main character, Simon of Cyrene, on a journey which transforms his life, and that of the reader, from one of despair and defeat to success and triumph!

(hardcover)　ISBN 091498473X　**$14.95**

Home Business Happiness　　　—Cheri Fuller

Subtitled: *Secrets On Keeping The Family Ship Afloat From Entrepreneurs Who Made It*. More than 26 million people in the US work at home businesses. *Home Business Happiness* is your network for success! In a reader-friendly style, Author Cheri Fuller offers valuable advice from some of the most inventive and pioneering entrepreneurs in the country. Some of the topics included are: Starting a Home Business, Time Management, and Avoiding Potential Pitfalls.

(trade paper)　ISBN 0914984705　**$12.95**

Migraine—Winning The Fight of Your Life　　　—Charles Theisler

This book describes the hurt, loneliness, and agony that migraine sufferers experience and the difficulty they must live with. It explains the different types of migraines and their symptoms, as well as the related health hazards. Gives 200 ways to help fight off migraines, and shows how to experience fewer headaches, reduce their duration, and decrease the agony and pain involved.

(trade paper)　ISBN 0914984632　**$10.95**

Books by Starburst Publishers—cont'd

Parenting With Respect and Peacefulness —Louise A. Dietzel

Subtitled: *The Most Difficult Job in the World*. Parents who love and respect themselves parent with respect and peaceful-ness. Yet, parenting with respect is the most difficult job in the world. This book informs parents that respect and peace communicate love—creating an atmosphere for children to maximize their development as they feel loved, valued, and safe. Parents learn authority and control by a common sense approach to day-to-day situations in parenting.

(trade paper) ISBN 0914984667 **$10.95**

A Woman's Guide To Spiritual Power —Nancy L. Dorner

Subtitled: *Through Scriptural Prayer*. Do your prayers seem to go "against a brick wall"? Does God sometimes seem far away or non-existent? If your answer is "Yes," you are not alone. Prayer must be the cornerstone of your relationship to God. "This book is a powerful tool for anyone who is serious about prayer and discipleship." —Florence Littauer

(trade paper) ISBN 0914984470 **$9.95**

Purchasing Information:

Books are available from your favorite bookstore, either from current stock or special order. To assist bookstore in locating your selection be sure to give title, author, and ISBN #. If unable to purchase from the bookstore you may order direct from STARBURST PUBLISHERS. When ordering enclose full payment plus $3.00 for shipping and handling ($4.00 if Canada or Overseas). Payment in US Funds only. Please allow two to three weeks minimum (longer overseas) for delivery. Make checks payable to and mail to STARBURST PUBLISHERS, P.O. Box 4123, LANCASTER, PA 17604. Credit card orders may also be placed by calling 1-800-441-1456 (credit card orders only), Mon-Fri, 8:30 a.m. – 5:30 p.m. Eastern Time. **Prices subject to change without notice.** Catalog available for a 9 x 12 self-addressed envelope with 4 first-class stamps.   10-97